Girl. You've Got This!

150 Workouts
For Every Day

2021

N. Rey | darebee.com

First Printing, 2021.
ISBN 13: 978-1-84481-178-6
ISBN 10: 1-84481-178-6

Published by New Line Books, London

Warning and Disclaimer
Although every precaution has been taken to verify the accuracy of the information contained herein, the author and
publisher assume no responsibility for any errors or omissions. No liability is assumed for damage or injury that may
result from the use of information contained within.

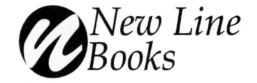

Author Bio

Neila Rey is the founder of Darebee, a global fitness resource. She is committed to democratizing fitness by removing the barriers to it and increasing accessibility. Every workout published in her books utilizes the latest in exercise science and has undergone thorough field testing and refinement through Darebee volunteers. When she's not busy running Darebee she is focused on finding fresh ways to make exercise easier and more enjoyable.

Thank you!

Thank you for purchasing 100 No-Equipment Workouts Vol. 3, DAREBEE project print edition. DAREBEE is a non-profit global fitness resource dedicated to making fitness accessible for everyone, no matter their circumstances. The project is supported exclusively via user donations and paperback royalties.

After printing costs and store fees every book developed by the DAREBEE project makes $1 and it goes directly into our project maintenance and development fund.

Each sale helps us keep the DAREBEE resource growing, maintain it and keep it up. Thank you for making a difference in its future!

Other books in this series include:

100 No-Equipment Workouts Vol 1.
100 No-Equipment Workouts Vol 2.
100 No-Equipment Workouts Vol 3.
100 No-Equipment Workouts Vol 4.
100 Office Workouts
Pocket Workouts: 100 no-equipment workouts
ABS 100 Workouts: Visual Easy-To-Follow ABS Exercise Routines for All Fitness Levels
100 HIIT Workouts: Visual easy-to-follow routines for all fitness levels

Index

Index

The Manual

Workout posters are read from left to right and contain the following information: grid with exercises (images), number of reps (repetitions) next to each, number of sets for your fitness level (I, II or III) and rest time.

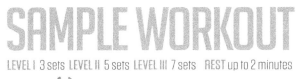

LEVEL I 3 sets LEVEL II 5 sets LEVEL III 7 sets REST up to 2 minutes

Difficulty Levels:

Level I: normal

Level II: hard

Level III: advanced

10 jumping jack

20 high knees

20 punches

one squat

20 lunges

10-count plank hold

20 climbers

10 plank jump-ins

to failure push-ups

1 set

10 jumping jacks

20 high knees (10 each leg)

20 punches (10 each arm)

one squat = 1 squat

20 lunges (10 each leg)

10-count plank (hold while counting to 10)

20 climbers (10 each leg)

10 plank jump-ins

to failure push-ups (your maximum)

Up to 2 minutes rest between sets

30 seconds, 60 seconds or 2 minutes - it's up to you.

"Reps" stands for repetitions, how many times an exercise is performed. Reps are usually located next to each exercise's name. Number of reps is always a total number for both legs / arms / sides. It's easier to count this way: e.g. if it says 20 climbers, it means that both legs are already counted in - it is 10 reps each leg.

Reps to failure means to muscle failure = your personal maximum, you repeat the move until you can't. It can be anything from one rep to twenty, normally applies to more challenging exercises. The goal is to do as many as you possibly can.

The transition from exercise to exercise is an important part of each circuit (set) - it is often what makes a particular workout more effective. Transitions are carefully worked out to hyperload specific muscle groups more for better results. For example if you see a plank followed by push-ups it means that you start performing push-ups right after you finished with the plank avoiding dropping your body on the floor in between.

There is no rest between exercises - only after sets, unless specified otherwise. You have to complete the entire set going from one exercise to the next as fast as you can before you can rest.

What does "up to 2 minutes rest" mean: it means you can rest for up to 2 minutes but the sooner you can go again the better. Eventually your recovery time will improve naturally, you won't need all two minutes to recover - and that will also be an indication of your improving fitness.

Recommended rest time:

Level I: 2 minutes or less
Level II: 60 seconds or less
Level III: 30 seconds or less

You can start with a single individual workout from the collection and see how you feel. If you are new to bodyweight training always start any workout on Level I (level of difficulty).

You can pick any number of workouts per week, usually between 3 and 5 and rotate them for maximum results.

Video Exercise Library: http://darebee.com/video

*I already know
what giving up feels like.
I want to see what happens
if I don't.*

Neila Rey

#1

Adira Workout

ADIRA

DAREBEE WORKOUT © darebee.com

LEVEL I 3 sets **LEVEL II** 5 sets **LEVEL III** 7 sets **REST** up to 2 minutes

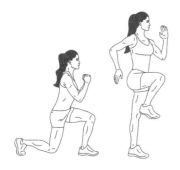

6 lunge step-ups

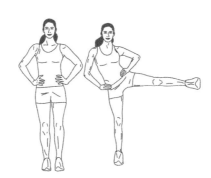

10 side leg raises

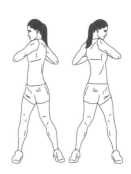

6 torso twists

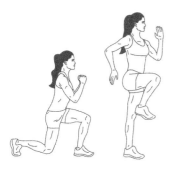

6 lunge step-ups

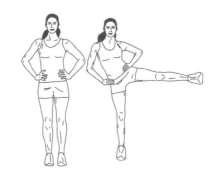

10 side leg raises

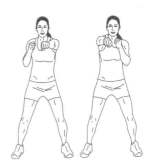

10 punches

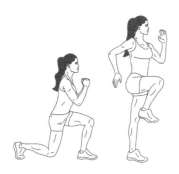

6 lunge step-ups

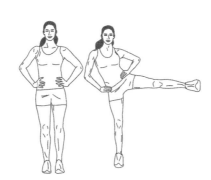

10 side leg raises

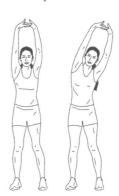

6 side bends

#2

Amazon Workout

AMAZON

DAREBEE WORKOUT © darebee.com

LEVEL I 3 sets **LEVEL II** 5 sets **LEVEL III** 7 sets **REST** up to 2 minutes

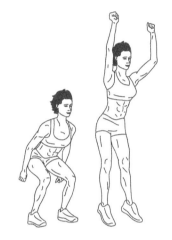

2 jump squats

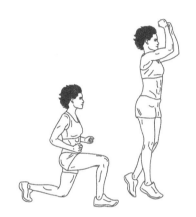

10 jumping lunges

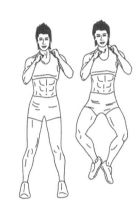

2 hop heel clicks

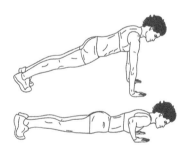

10 push-ups

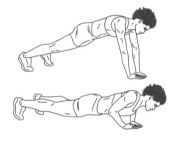

2 close grip push-ups

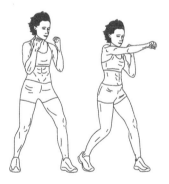

20 punches

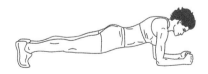

10-count elbow plank

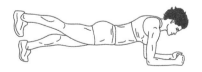

20-count raised leg plank

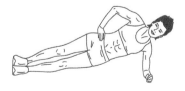

20-count side plank

#3

Andromeda Workout

Andromeda

DAREBEE WORKOUT © darebee.com

LEVEL I 3 sets **LEVEL II** 5 sets **LEVEL III** 7 sets **REST** up to 2 minutes

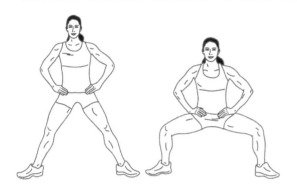

10 wide squats

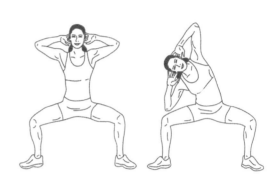

10 squat hold side bends

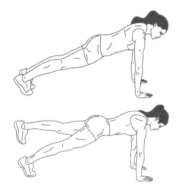

10 plank leg raises

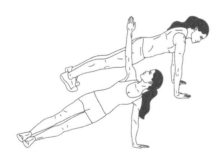

10 plank rotations

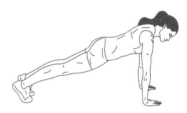

10-count plank hold

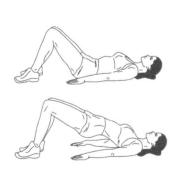

10 bridges

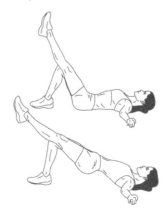

4 single leg bridges

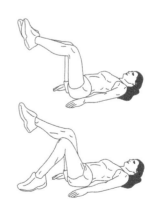

10 toe taps

#4

Anthem Workout

ANTHEM

DAREBEE WORKOUT © darebee.com

LEVEL I 3 sets **LEVEL II** 5 sets **LEVEL III** 7 sets **REST** up to 2 minutes

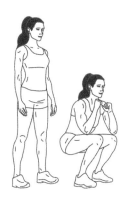

4 squats

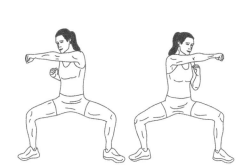

20 squat hold punches

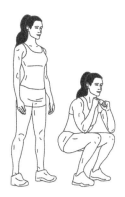

4 squats

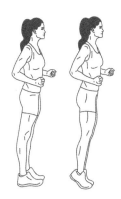

4 calf raises

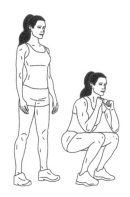

4 squats

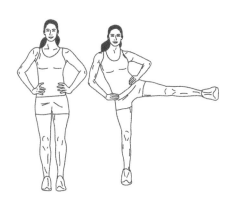

20 side leg raises

#5

Aphrodite Workout

Aphrodite

DAREBEE WORKOUT © darebee.com

LEVEL I 3 sets **LEVEL II** 5 sets **LEVEL III** 7 sets

2 minutes rest between sets

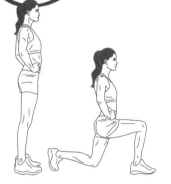

20 lunges

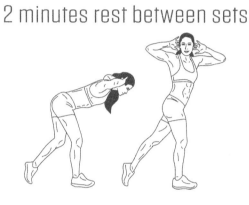

10 deadlift & twist

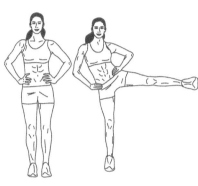

20 side leg raises

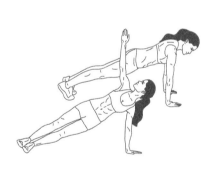

20 plank rotations

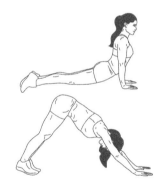

10 downward upward dog

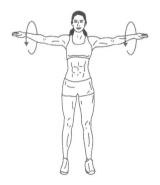

20 raised arm circles

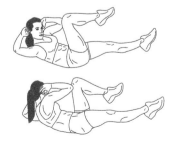

20 knee-to-elbow

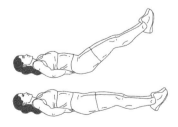

10 leg raises

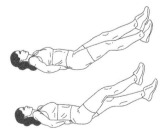

20 scissors

#6

Artemis Workout

NOTES

Artemis

DAREBEE WORKOUT © darebee.com
LEVEL I 3 sets LEVEL II 5 sets LEVEL III 7 sets
REST up to 2 minutes

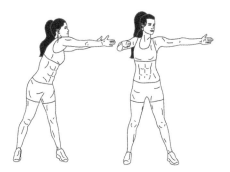

20 archers

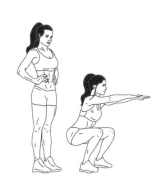

2 squats

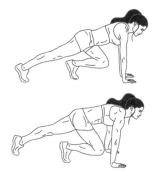

20 climbers

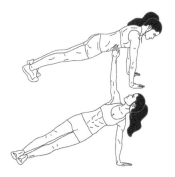

2 planks w/ rotations

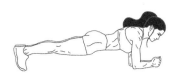

10-count elbow plank

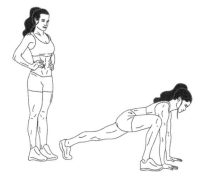

10 deep lunges

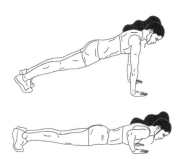

2 push-ups

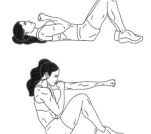

10 sit-up punches

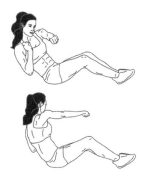

10 sititing punches

#7

Atalanta Workout

Atalanta

DAREBEE WORKOUT © darebee.com

LEVEL I 3 sets **LEVEL II** 5 sets **LEVEL III** 7 sets **REST** up to 2 minutes

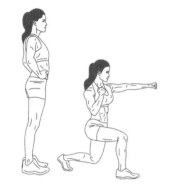

20 lunge punches

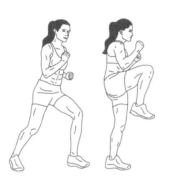

20 knee strikes

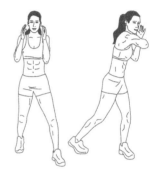

20 elbow strikes

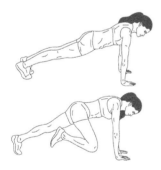

20 slow climbers

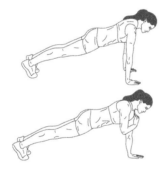

20 shoulder taps

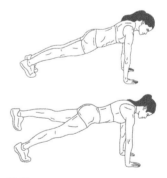

20 plank leg raises

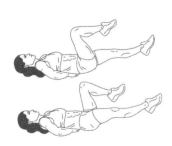

10 bicycle crunches

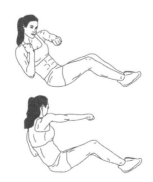

10 sitting punches

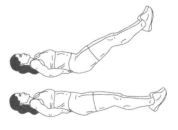

10 leg raises

#8

Athena Workout

ATHENA

DAREBEE WORKOUT © darebee.com

LEVEL I 3 sets **LEVEL II** 5 sets **LEVEL III** 7 sets **REST** up to 2 minutes

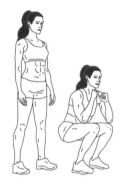
4 squats

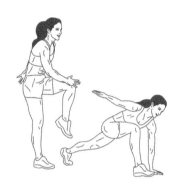
10 knee tap reverse lunges

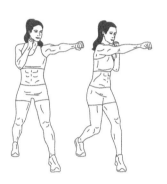
20 punches

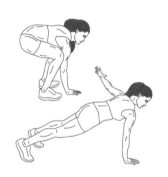
4 one-arm plank jump-ins

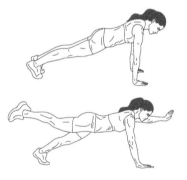
4 alt arm/leg plank

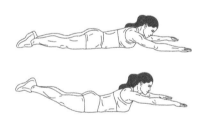
4 supergirl stretch

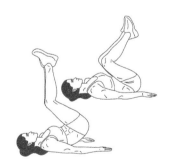
10 reverse crunches

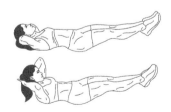
4 raised leg crunches

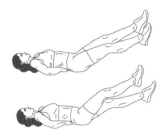
10 scissors

#9

Banshee Workout

BANSHEE

DAREBEE WORKOUT © darebee.com

LEVEL I 3 sets **LEVEL II** 4 sets **LEVEL III** 5 sets **REST** up to 2 minutes

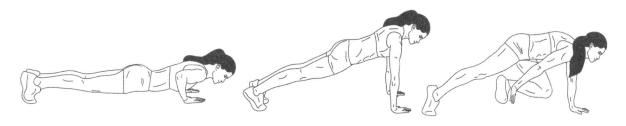

10combos push-up + climber tap (each foot)

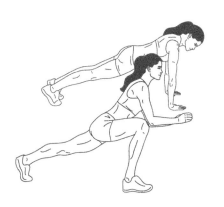

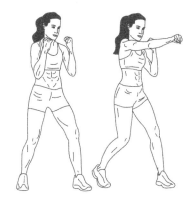

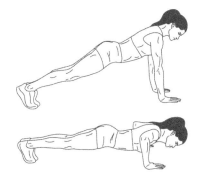

4 plank into lunges   **20** punches   **4** wide grip push-ups

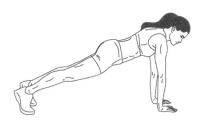

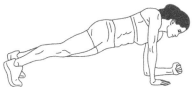

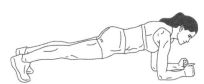

4 up and down planks

#10

Beast Mode Workout

BEAST MODE

DAREBEE WORKOUT
ⓒ darebee.com
up to 2 minutes
rest between exercises

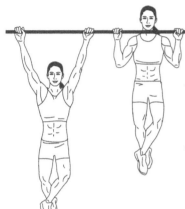

to failure
pull-ups
4 sets in total
30 seconds rest

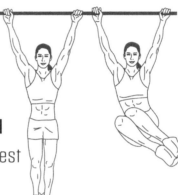

to failure
knee-up twists
4 sets in total
30 seconds rest

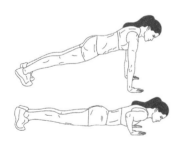

to failure
push-ups
4 sets in total
30 seconds rest

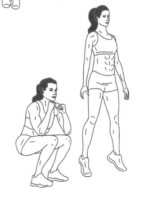

to failure
jump squats
4 sets in total
30 seconds rest

to failure elbow plank hold
in one go

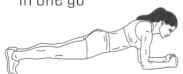

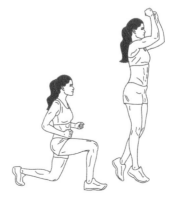

to failure
jumping lunges
4 sets in total
30 seconds rest

#11

Boudicca Workout

BOUDICCA

DAREBEE WORKOUT © darebee.com

LEVEL I 3 sets **LEVEL II** 5 sets **LEVEL III** 7 sets **REST** up to 2 minutes

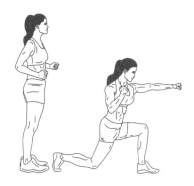

20 lunge punches

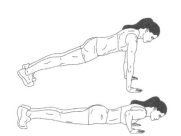

10 push-ups

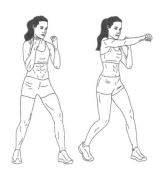

20 punches

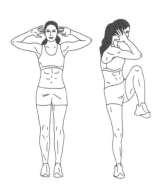

20 knee-to-elbows

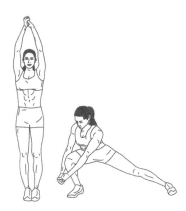

10 deep cross chops

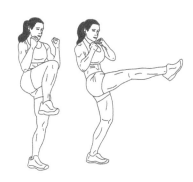

20 front kicks

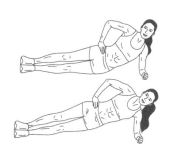

20 side bridges

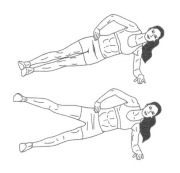

10 side plank leg raises

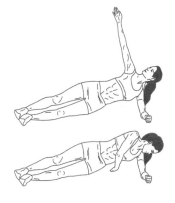

20 side plank rotations

#12

Bright & Beautiful Workout

Bright & Beautiful

DAREBEE WORKOUT © darebee.com

LEVEL I 3 sets **LEVEL II** 5 sets **LEVEL III** 7 sets **REST** up to 2 minutes

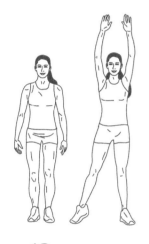

10 step jacks

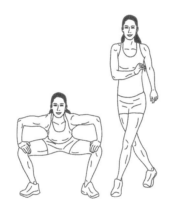

6 squat step backs

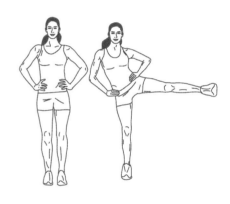

10 side leg raises

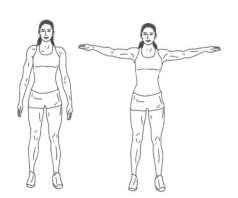

20 arm raises

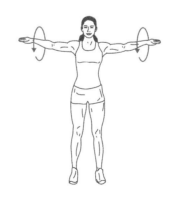

20 raised arm circles

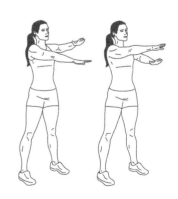

20 arm scissors

#13

Callisto Workout

Callisto

DAREBEE WORKOUT © darebee.com

LEVEL I 3 sets **LEVEL II** 5 sets **LEVEL III** 7 sets **REST** up to 2 minutes

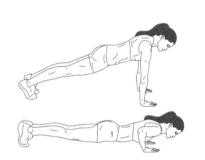

10 push-ups

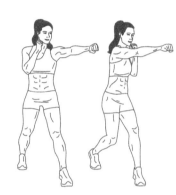

20 punches

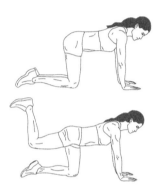

10 donkey kicks

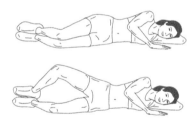

10 clamshells

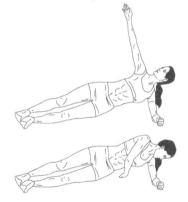

10 side planks rotations

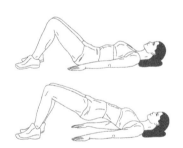

10 bridges

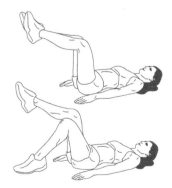

10 toe taps

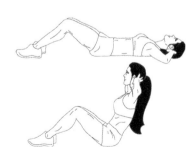

10 sit-ups

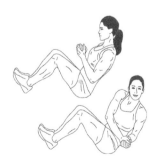

10 sitting twists

#14

Can & Will Workout

I CAN & I WILL

DAREBEE WORKOUT © darebee.com

LEVEL I 3 sets **LEVEL II** 5 sets **LEVEL III** 7 sets **REST** up to 2 minutes

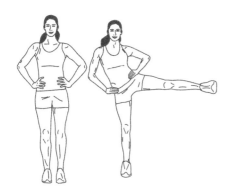

20 side leg raises

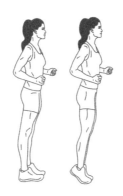

5 calf raises

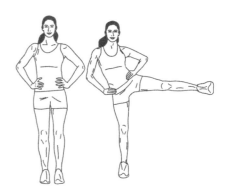

20 side leg raises

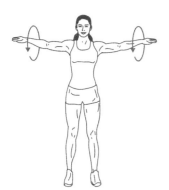

20 arm circles

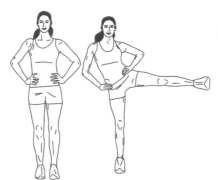

20 side leg raises

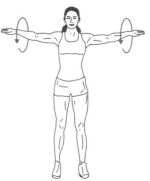

20 arm circles

#15

Chimera Workout

CHIMERA

DAREBEE WORKOUT © darebee.com

LEVEL I 3 sets **LEVEL II** 5 sets **LEVEL III** 7 sets **REST** up to 2 minutes

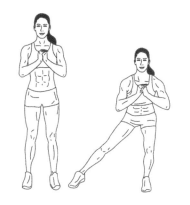

20 side-to-side lunges

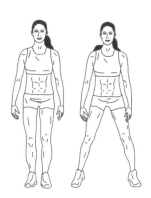

20combos half jack + side leg raise

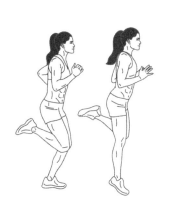

10 butt kicks

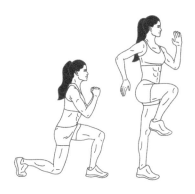

10 lunge step-ups

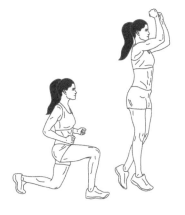

10 jumping lunges

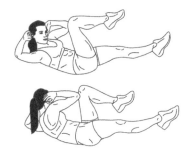

10 knee-to-elbow crunches

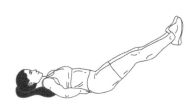

10-count raised leg hold

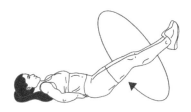

10 raised leg circles

#16

Chosen One Workout

CHOSEN ONE

DAREBEE WORKOUT © darebee.com

LEVEL I 3 sets **LEVEL II** 5 sets **LEVEL III** 7 sets **REST** up to 2 minutes

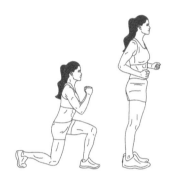

8 reverse lunges

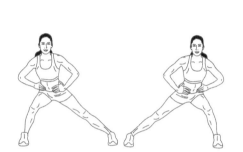

4 side-to-side lunges

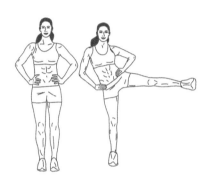

20 side leg raises

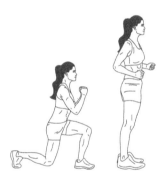

8 reverse lunges

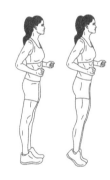

4 calf raises

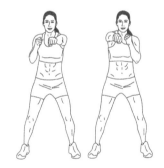

20 punches

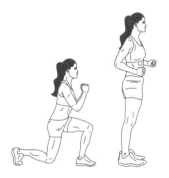

8 reverse lunges

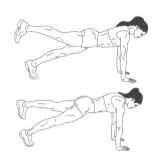

4 plank leg raises

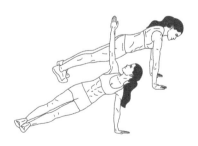

8 plank rotations

#17

Druid Workout

DRUID

DAREBEE WORKOUT © darebee.com

LEVEL I 3 sets **LEVEL II** 5 sets **LEVEL III** 7 sets **REST** up to 2 minutes

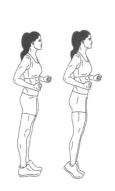

6 calf raises

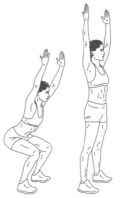

10 high squats

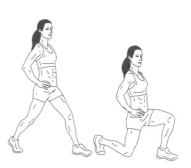

6 split lunges

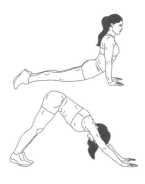

6 downward upward dogs

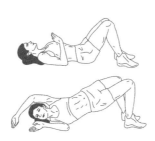

10 bridge taps

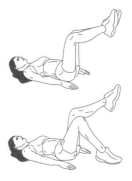

6 toe taps

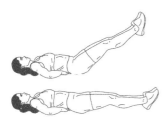

6 leg raises

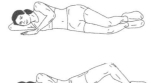

10 clamshells

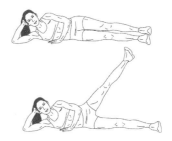

6 side leg raises

#18

Empress Workout

THE EMPRESS

DAREBEE WORKOUT © darebee.com

LEVEL I 3 sets **LEVEL II** 5 sets **LEVEL III** 7 sets **REST** up to 2 minutes

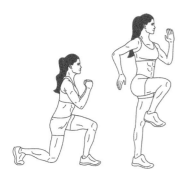

20 lunge step-ups

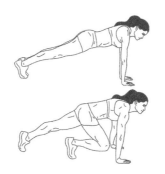

20 slow climbers

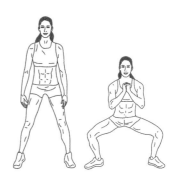

20 wide squats

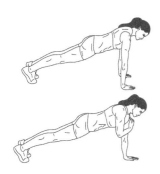

20 shoulder taps

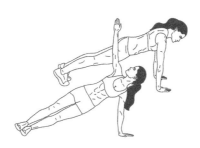

10 plank rotations

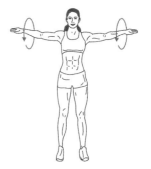

20 raised arm circles

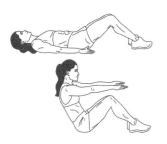

10 sit-ups

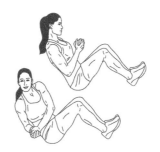

10 sitting twists

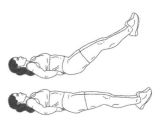

10 leg raises

#19

Epic Glutes Workout

EPIC GLUTES

WORKOUT by DAREBEE © darebee.com

3 sets | 2 minutes rest

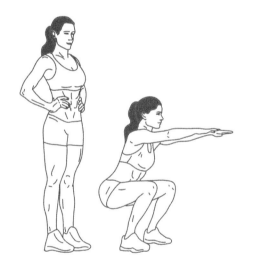
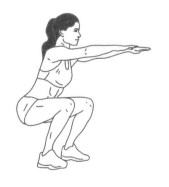

5 squats

5-count squat hold

5 squats

5-count squat hold

5 squats

5-count squat hold

5 squats

5-count squat hold

5 squats

5-count squat hold

#20

Femme Fatale Workout

FEMME FATALE

DAREBEE
WORKOUT
© darebee.com
LEVEL I 3 sets
LEVEL II 5 sets
LEVEL III 7 sets
2 minutes rest

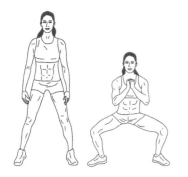

10 goblet squats

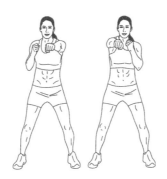

20 punches

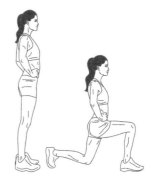

10 lunges

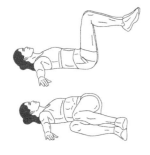

10 half wipers

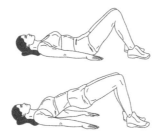

10 bridges

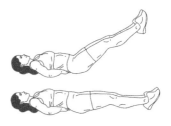

10 leg raises

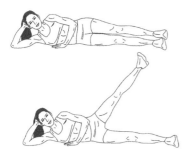

20 side leg raises

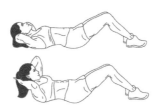

20 crunches

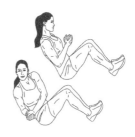

20 sitting twists

#21

Fierce Workout

FIERCE

DAREBEE WORKOUT © darebee.com

LEVEL I 3 sets **LEVEL II** 5 sets **LEVEL III** 7 sets **REST** up to 2 minutes

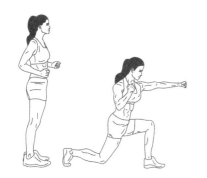

10 lunge punches

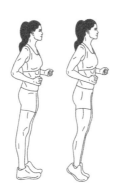

10 calf raises

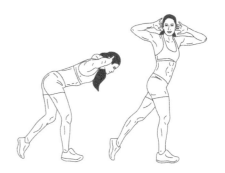

10 deadlift & twist

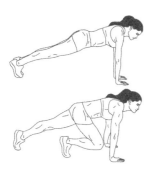

6 slow climbers

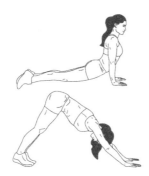

6 downward upward dog

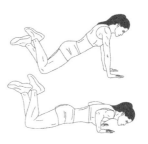

6 knee push-ups

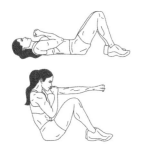

6 sit-up punches

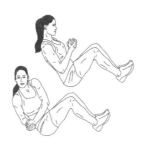

6 sitting twists

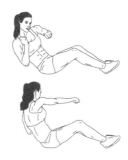

6 sitting punches

#22

Filler Workout

5-MINUTE
FILLER

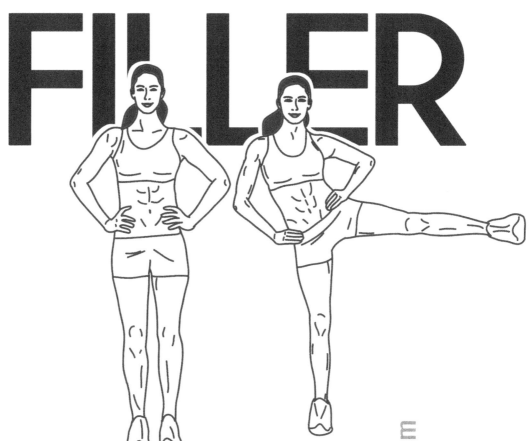

30 side leg raises (right leg)

30 side leg raises (left leg)

60 seconds rest

30 side leg raises (right leg)

30 side leg raises (left leg)

60 seconds rest

30 side leg raises (right leg)

30 side leg raises (left leg)

done

#23

Girl Who Dared Workout

THE GIRL WHO DARED

DAREBEE WORKOUT © darebee.com

LEVEL I 3 sets **LEVEL II** 5 sets **LEVEL III** 7 sets **REST** up to 2 minutes

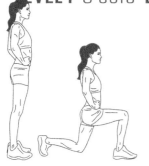

10 lunges

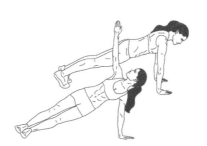

4 plank rotations

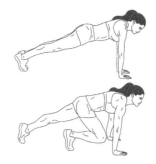

10 slow climbers

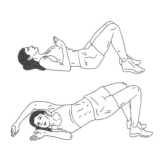

10 bridge taps

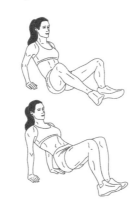

4 butterfly dips

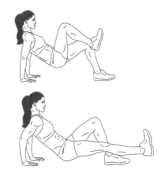

10 raised front kicks

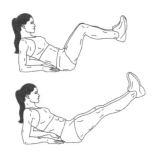

10 crunch kicks

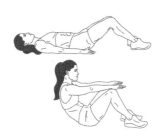

4 sit-ups

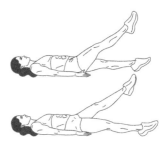

10 flutter kicks

#24

Glutes, Quads, Hamstrings & Calves Workout

Glutes, Quads, Hamstrings, & Calves

workout by DAREBEE
© darebee.com

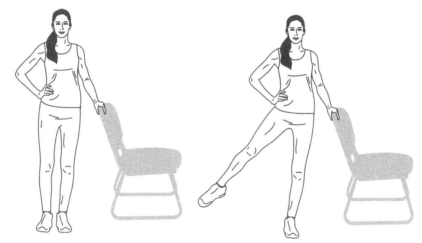

40 side leg raises

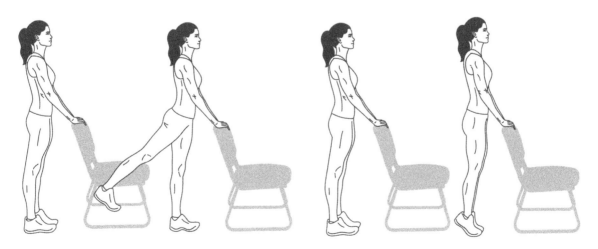

40 back kicks   **40** calf raises

#25

Gone Wild Workout

NOTES

GONE WILD

DAREBEE WORKOUT © darebee.com

LEVEL I 3 sets **LEVEL II** 5 sets **LEVEL III** 7 sets **REST** up to 2 minutes

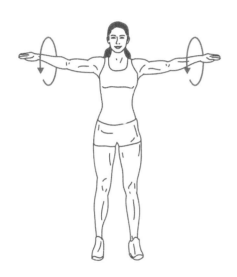

10 raised arm circles

6 arm scissors

10 raised arm circles

6 arm scissors

10 raised arm circles

6 arm scissors

10 raised arm circles

6 arm scissors

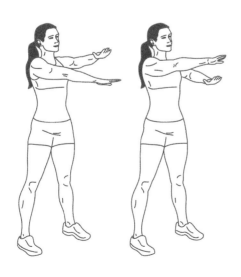

#26

Healer Workout

HEALER

DAREBEE WORKOUT © darebee.com

LEVEL I 3 sets **LEVEL II** 5 sets **LEVEL III** 7 sets **REST** up to 2 minutes

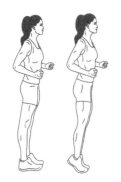

5 calf raises

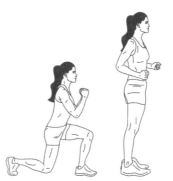

10 reverse lunges

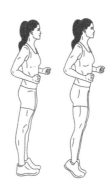

5 calf raises

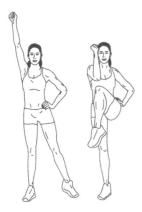

10 knee-to-elbows

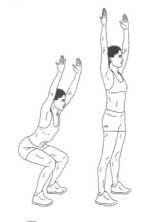

5 high squats

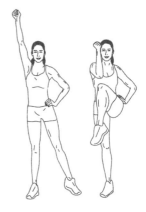

10 knee-to-elbows

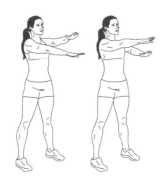

10 arm scissors

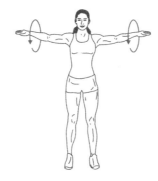

10 raised arm circles

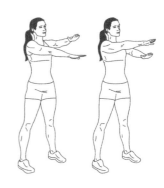

10 arm scissors

#27

Holistic Workout

HOLISTIC

DAREBEE WORKOUT © darebee.com

5 sets | 2 minutes rest between sets

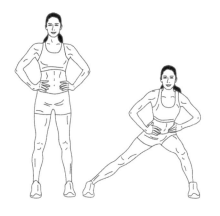

20 side lunges

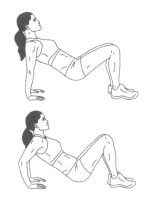

10 tricep dips

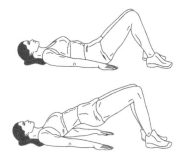

20 bridges

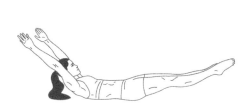

20-count hollow hold

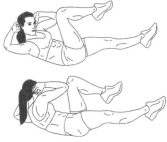

10 knee-to-elbow crunches

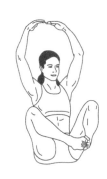

20-count O-pose hold

#28

Home Upperbody Tone Workout

HOME UPPERBODY TONE

DAREBEE WORKOUT
© darebee.com
Level I   3 sets
Level II   4 sets
Level III 5 sets
2 minutes rest

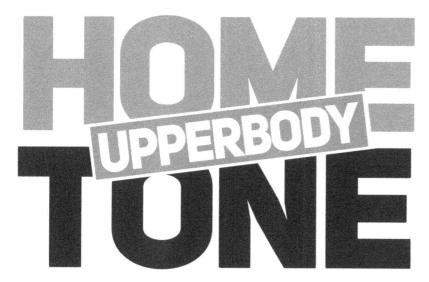

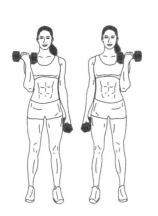

20 alternating bicep curls

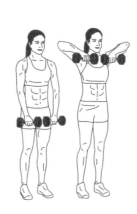

10 upright rows

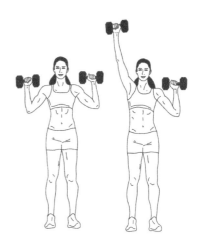

10 alternating shoulder press

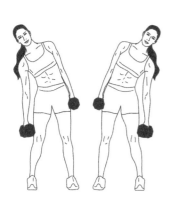

10 side bends

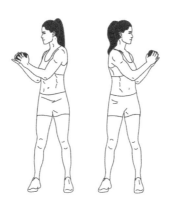

10 core twists

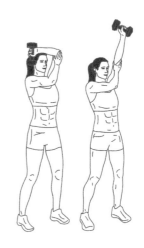

20 tricep extensions

#29

Huntress Workout

HUNTRESS

DAREBEE WORKOUT © darebee.com

LEVEL I 3 sets **LEVEL II** 5 sets **LEVEL III** 7 sets **REST** up to 2 minutes

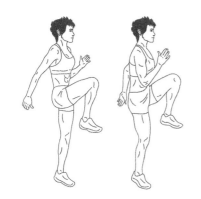

20 high knees

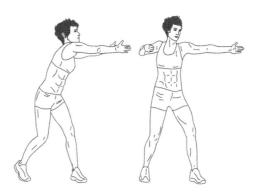

20 archers

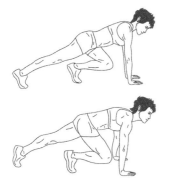

10 climbers

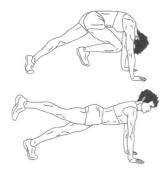

10 knee-in kick backs

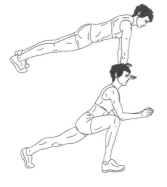

10 plank into lunges

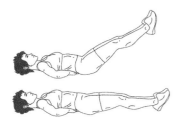

10 leg raises

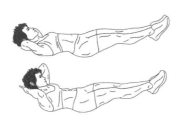

10 raised legs crunches

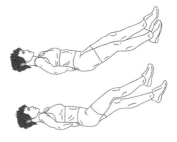

10 scissors

#30

Imp Workout

NOTES

IMP

DAREBEE WORKOUT © darebee.com

LEVEL I 3 sets **LEVEL II** 5 sets **LEVEL III** 7 sets **REST** up to 2 minutes

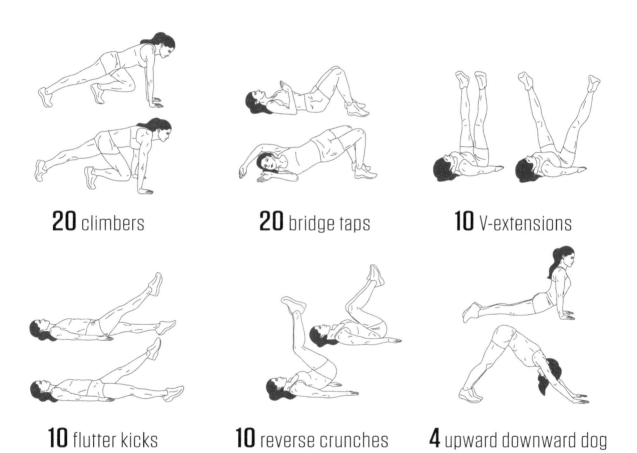

20 climbers   **20** bridge taps   **10** V-extensions

10 flutter kicks   **10** reverse crunches   **4** upward downward dog

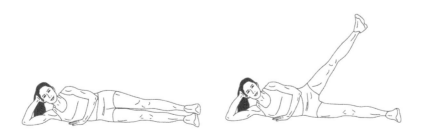

20 side leg raises

#31

Ironheart Workout

IRONHEART

DAREBEE WORKOUT © darebee.com

LEVEL I 3 sets **LEVEL II** 5 sets **LEVEL III** 7 sets **REST** up to 2 minutes

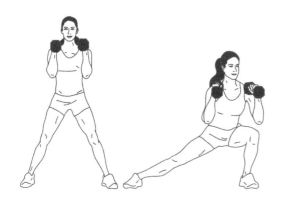

12 side lunges

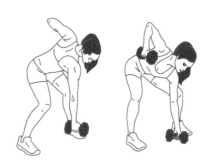

12 alternating bent over rows

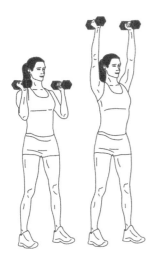

6 shoulder press

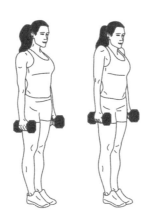

6 shrugs

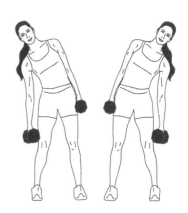

12 side bends

#32

Iron Maiden Workout

IRON MAIDEN

DAREBEE WORKOUT © darebee.com

LEVEL I 3 sets **LEVEL II** 4 sets **LEVEL III** 5 sets **REST** up to 2 minutes

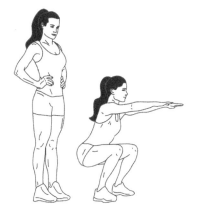

20 squats

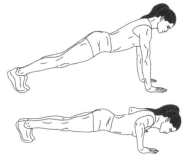

4 push-ups

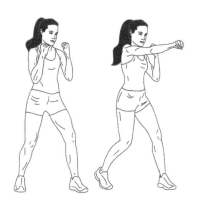

20 punches

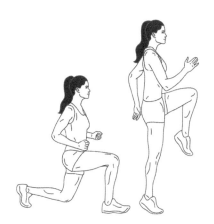

20 lunge step-ups

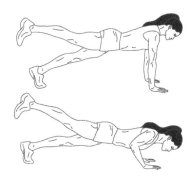

4 raised leg push-ups

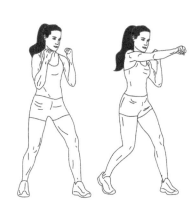

20 punches

#33

Keeper Workout

KEEPER

DAREBEE WORKOUT © darebee.com

LEVEL I 3 sets **LEVEL II** 5 sets **LEVEL III** 7 sets **REST** up to 2 minutes

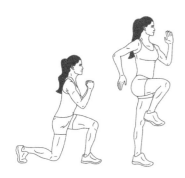

4 lunge step-ups

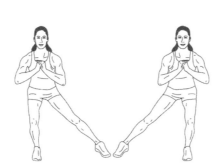

4 side-to-side lunges

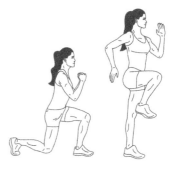

4 lunge step-ups

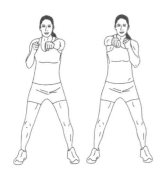

20 punches

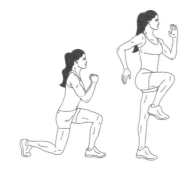

4 lunge step-ups

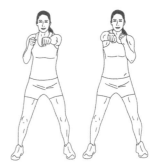

20 punches

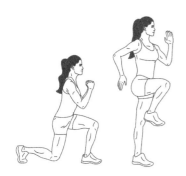

4 lunge step-ups

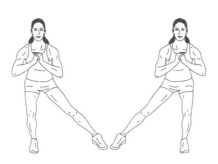

4 side-to-side lunges

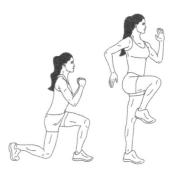

4 lunge step-ups

#34

Lift & Tone Workout

lift & tone

DAREBEE WORKOUT © darebee.com

2 minutes rest between exercises

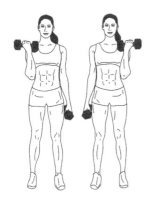

20 alt bicep curls
x 4 sets in total
20 seconds rest
between sets

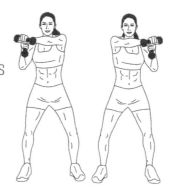

20 punches
x 4 sets in total
20 seconds rest
between sets

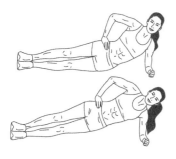

20 side bridges
x 4 sets in total
20 seconds rest
between sets

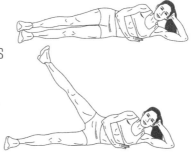

20 side leg raises
x 4 sets in total
20 seconds rest
between sets

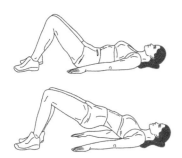

20 bridges
x 4 sets in total
20 seconds rest
between sets

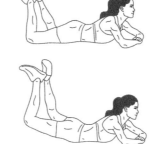

20 glute flex
x 4 sets in total
20 seconds rest
between sets

#35

Morrigan Workout

MORRIGAN

DAREBEE WORKOUT © darebee.com

LEVEL I 3 sets **LEVEL II** 5 sets **LEVEL III** 7 sets **REST** up to 2 minutes

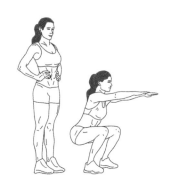

20 squats

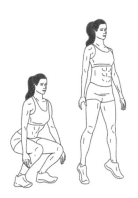

10 jump squats

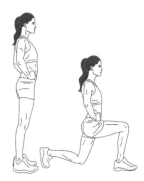

20 lunges

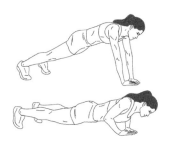

2 close grip push-ups

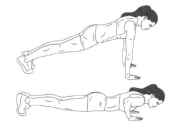

2 classic grip push-ups

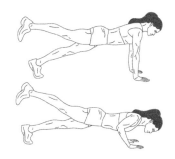

4 raised leg push-ups

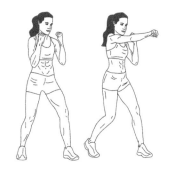

40 punches

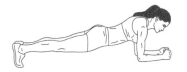

20sec elbow plank

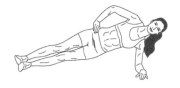

40sec side elbow plank

#36

New Me Workout

this is the
new me

DAREBEE WORKOUT © darebee.com

LEVEL I 3 sets **LEVEL II** 5 sets **LEVEL III** 7 sets **REST** up to 2 minutes

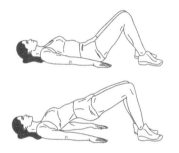

10 bridges

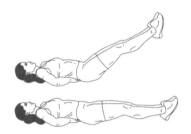

10 leg raises

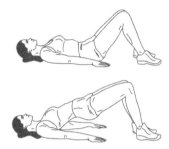

10 bridges

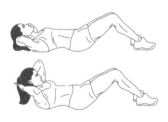

10 crunches

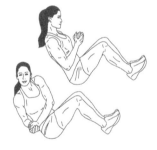

10 sitting twists

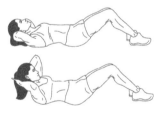

10 crunches

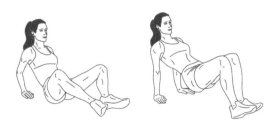

10 butterfly dips

#37

Power 10 Workout

Power 10

DAREBEE WORKOUT © darebee.com
3 sets | 60 seconds rest between sets

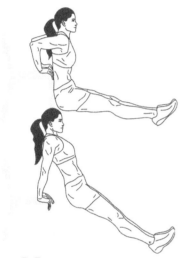

20 tricep dips

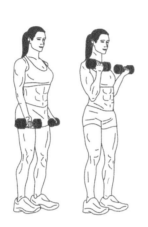

20 bicep curls

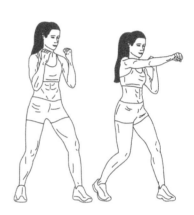

20 punches

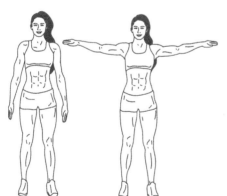

20 arm raises

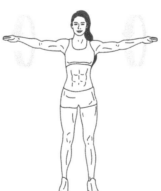

20 arm circles

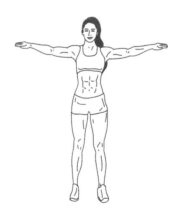

20sec raised arm hold

Don't have dumbbells? Use water bottles or cans of beans instead.
Keep your arms up between raised arm circles and raised arm hold.

#38

Power 18 Workout

Power **18**

DAREBEE WORKOUT © darebee.com

Use comfortable weights for this routine.
Pick up heavier weights the moment it gets easier.

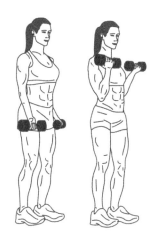

10 alt bicep curls
3 sets | 20 sec rest

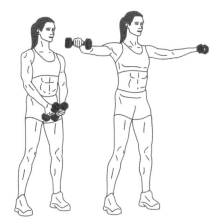

5 lateral raises
3 sets | 20 sec rest

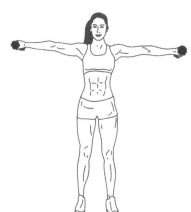

10-count hold
once

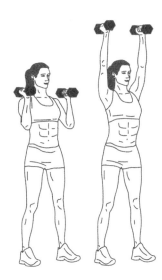

5 shoulder presses
3 sets | 20 sec rest

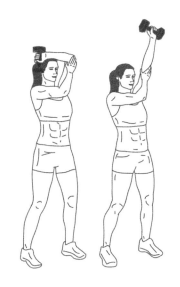

10 tricep extensions
3 sets | 20 sec rest

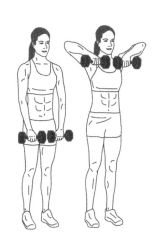

10 upright rows
3 sets | 20 sec rest

#39

Saber Workout

SABER

DAREBEE WORKOUT © darebee.com

LEVEL I 3 sets **LEVEL II** 5 sets **LEVEL III** 7 sets **REST** up to 2 minutes

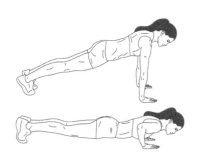

10 push-ups

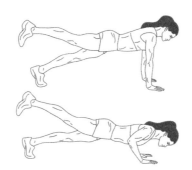

4 raised leg push-ups

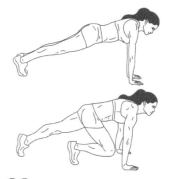

20 slow climbers

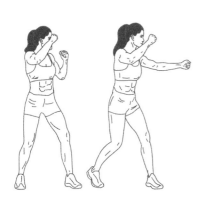

20 backfists

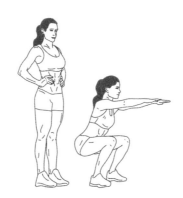

10 squats

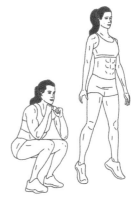

10 jump squats

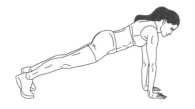
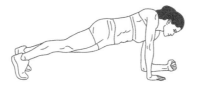
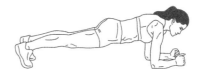

10 up and down planks

#40

Sculptor Plus Workout

SCULPTOR+

DAREBEE WORKOUT FOR ARMS, CHEST AND BACK
© darebee.com

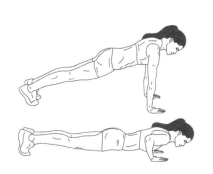
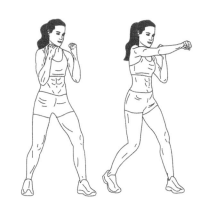

5 push-ups
20 punches
5 push-ups
20 punches
5 push-ups
20 punches
2 minutes rest

1kg / 2lb
dumbbells

go as fast as you can
non-stop

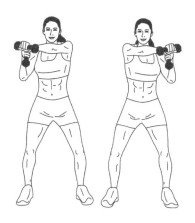

1 minute punches
1 minute rest
1 minute punches
2 minutes rest

5kg / 10lb
dumbbells

tip: use dumbbells
you can *just* curl
12 reps with

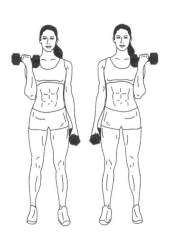

8 alt bicep curls
2 minutes rest
10 alt bicep curls
2 minutes rest
12 alt bicep curls
done

#41

Setting Goals Workout

Setting Goals

WORKOUT
BY DAREBEE
© darebee.com

Level I   3 sets
Level II   5 sets
Level III   7 sets
2 minutes rest

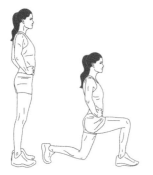

4 lunges

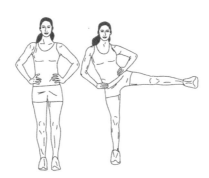

20 side leg raises

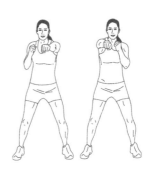

20 punches

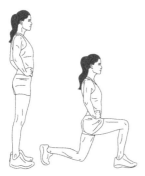

4 lunges

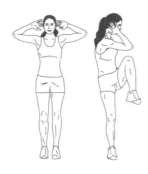

4 knee-to-elbows

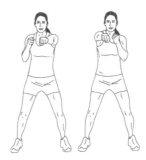

20 punches

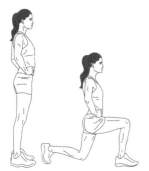

4 lunges

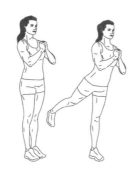

20 back leg raises

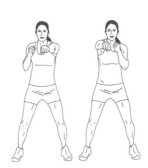

20 punches

#42

Spectacular Me Workout

spectacular
me

DAREBEE WORKOUT
© darebee.com

LEVEL I 3 sets **LEVEL II** 5 sets **LEVEL III** 7 sets **REST** up to 2 minutes

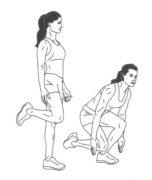

4 single leg squats

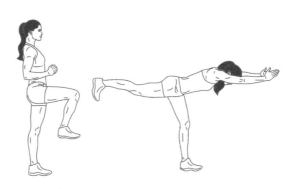

4 single leg deadlifts

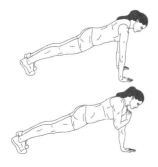

10 shoulder taps

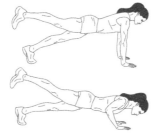

4 raised leg push-ups

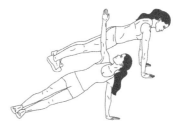

10 plank rotations

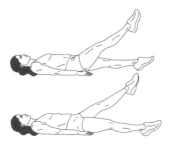

10 flutter kicks

#43

Stronger Today Workout

Stronger Today

DAREBEE WORKOUT © darebee.com
LEVEL I 3 sets LEVEL II 5 sets LEVEL III 7 sets
up to 2 minutes rest between sets

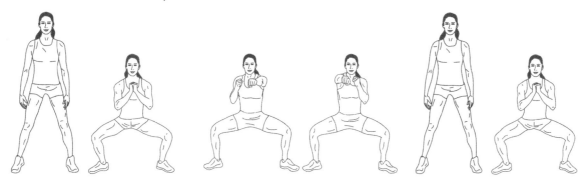

5 squats   **20** squat hold punches   **5** squats

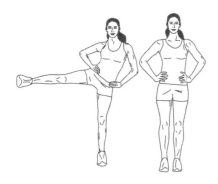
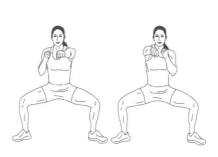
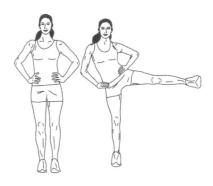

10 side leg raises
right leg

20 squat hold punches

10 side leg raises
left leg

#44

Take Charge Workout

TAKE CHARGE

DAREBEE WORKOUT
© darebee.com
LEVEL I 3 sets
LEVEL II 5 sets
LEVEL III 7 sets
REST up to 2 minutes

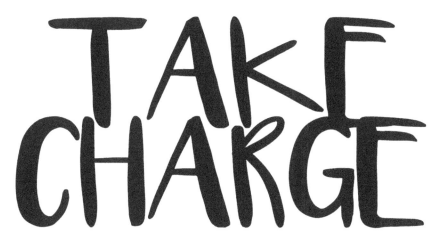

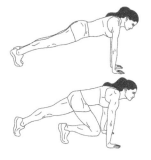
10 climbers

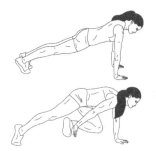
10 climber taps

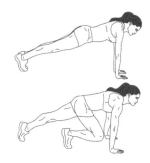
10 climbers

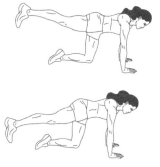
10 leg swings / left

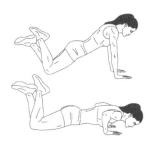
5 knee push-ups

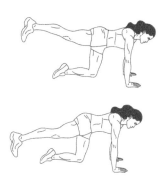
10 leg swings / right

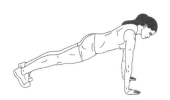
10-count plank hold

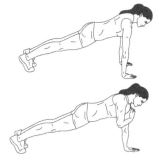
10 shoulder taps

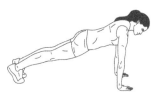
10-count plank hold

#45

Trim & Tone Arms Workout

TRIM & TONE
ARMS

WORKOUT
by DAREBEE
© darebee.com
2 minutes rest
between exercises

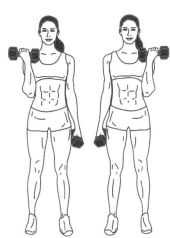

12 reps
x 5 sets
alternating bicep curls
20 seconds rest
between sets

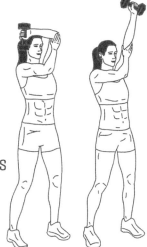

12 reps
x 5 sets
tricep extensions
20 seconds rest
between sets

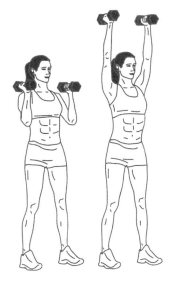

6 reps
x 5 sets
shoulder press
20 seconds rest
between sets

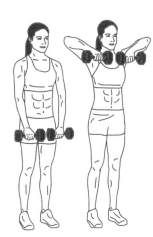

6 reps
x 5 sets
body rows
20 seconds rest
between sets

#46

Upperbody Blast Workout

UPPERBODY
BLAST

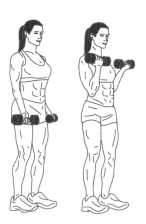

8 bicep curl
x 3 sets in total
20 seconds rest
between sets

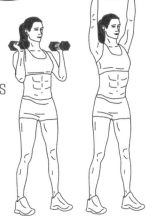

8 shoulder press
x 3 sets in total
20 seconds rest
between sets

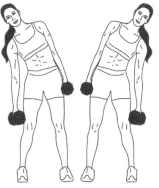

8 side-to-side tilts
x 3 sets in total
20 seconds rest
between sets

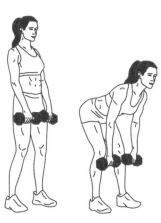

8 deadlifts
x 3 sets in total
20 seconds rest
between sets

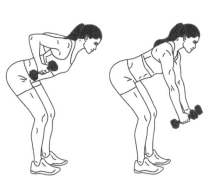

8 bent over rows
x 3 sets in total
20 seconds rest
between sets

#47

Valkyrie Workout

Valkyrìe

DAREBEE WORKOUT   © darebee.com

LEVEL I 3 sets   **LEVEL II** 5 sets   **LEVEL III** 7 sets   **REST** up to 2 minutes

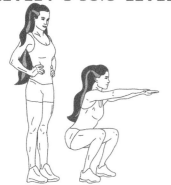

4 squats

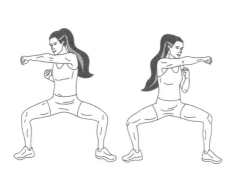

10 squat punches

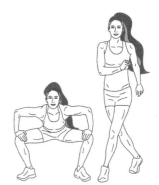

4 squat cross steps

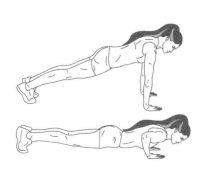

4 push-ups

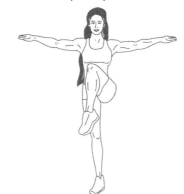

20-count balance stand

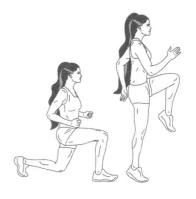

10 lunge step-ups

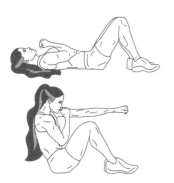

10 sit-up punches

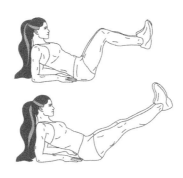

10 crunch kicks

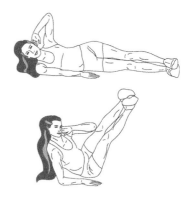

4 side Vs

#48

Vicious Workout

NOTES

VICIOUS

DAREBEE WORKOUT © darebee.com

LEVEL I 3 sets **LEVEL II** 5 sets **LEVEL III** 7 sets **REST** up to 2 minutes

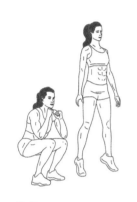

20 jump squats

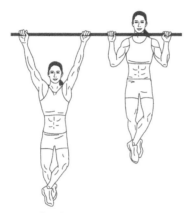

to failure pull-ups

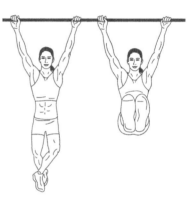

to failure leg raises

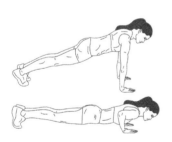

to failure push-ups

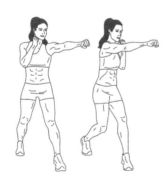

20 punches

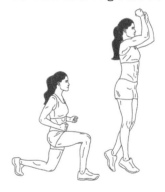

20 jumping lunges

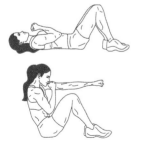

20 sit-up punches

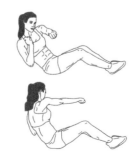

20 sitting punches

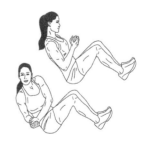

20 sitting twists

#49

Wasp Workout

THE WASP

DAREBEE WORKOUT © darebee.com

LEVEL I 3 sets **LEVEL II** 5 sets **LEVEL III** 7 sets **REST** up to 2 minutes

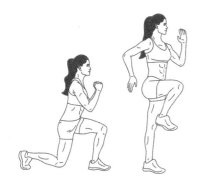

6 lunge step-ups

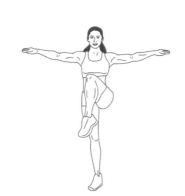

10-count balance hold (left)

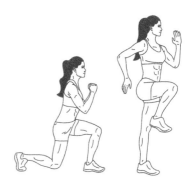

6 lunge step-ups

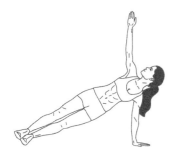

10-count side plank hold
left side

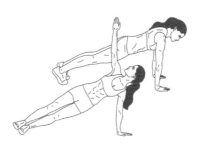

6 plank rotations

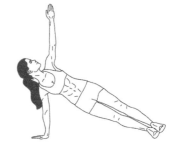

10-count side plank hold
right side

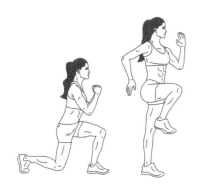

6 lunge step-ups

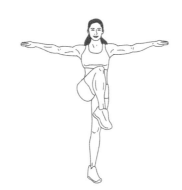

10-count balance hold (right)

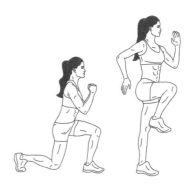

6 lunge step-ups

#50

Workout That Happened

WORKOUT THAT HAPPENED

BY DAREBEE © darebee.com

LEVEL I 3 sets **LEVEL II** 5 sets **LEVEL III** 7 sets **REST** up to 2 minutes

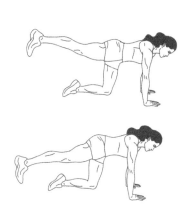

20 leg raises

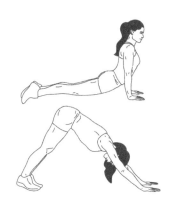

5 upward downward dog

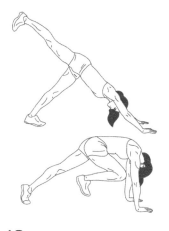

10 knee-in extensions

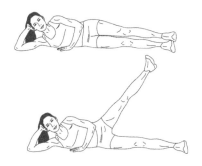

20 side leg raises

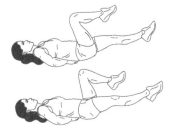

10 air bike crunches

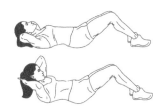

10 crunches

#51

Ace Workout

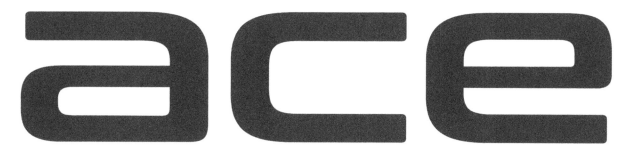

ace

DAREBEE WORKOUT © darebee.com

LEVEL I 3 sets **LEVEL II** 5 sets **LEVEL III** 7 sets **REST** up to 2 minutes

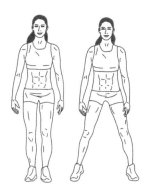

10 half jacks

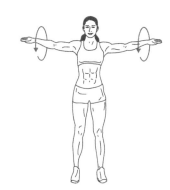

10 raised arm circles

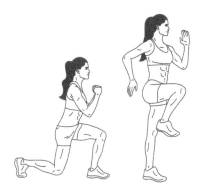

10 lunge step-ups

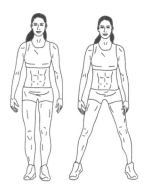

10 half jacks

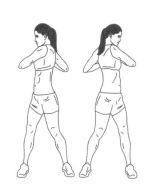

10 twists

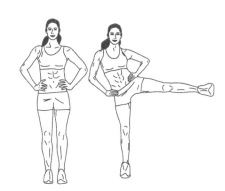

10 side leg raises

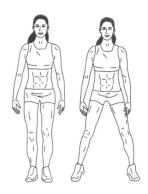

10 half jacks

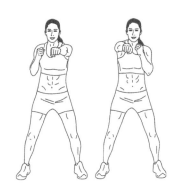

10 punches

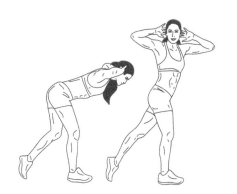

10 deadlift & twist

#52

Aloy Workout

Aloy

DAREBEE WORKOUT © darebee.com

LEVEL I 3 sets **LEVEL II** 5 sets **LEVEL III** 7 sets **REST** up to 2 minutes

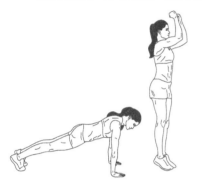

6 basic burpees w / jump

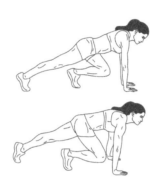

10 climbers

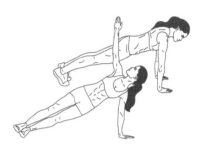

6 plank rotations

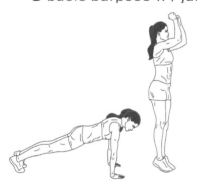

6 basic burpees w / jump

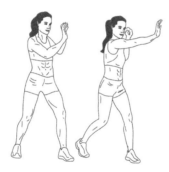

10 palm strikes

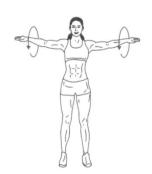

6 arm rotations

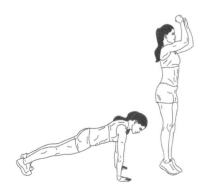

6 basic burpees w / jump

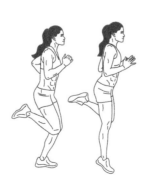

10 butt kicks

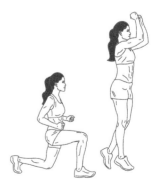

6 jumping lunges

#53

Aurora Workout

AURORA

DAREBEE WORKOUT © darebee.com

LEVEL I 3 sets **LEVEL II** 5 sets **LEVEL III** 7 sets **REST** up to 2 minutes

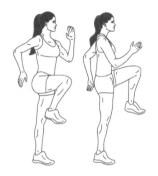

20 march steps

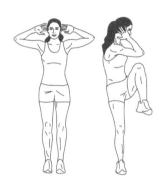

10 knee-to-elbows

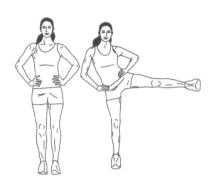

10 side leg raises

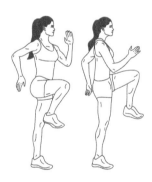

20 march steps

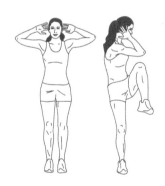

10 knee-to-elbows

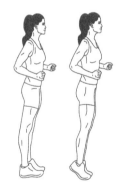

10 calf raises

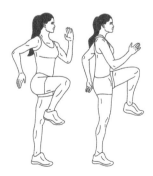

20 march steps

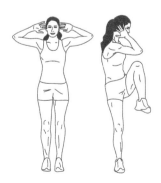

10 knee-to-elbows

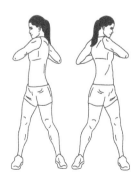

10 torso rotations

#54

Bellatrix Workout

Bellatrix

DAREBEE WORKOUT © darebee.com

LEVEL I 3 sets **LEVEL II** 5 sets **LEVEL III** 7 sets **REST** up to 2 minutes

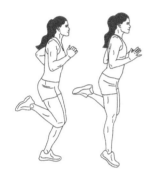

10 butt kicks

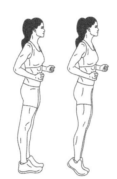

5 calf raises

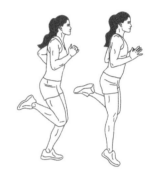

10 butt kicks

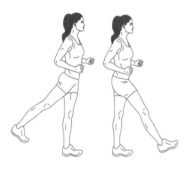

10 leg swings
left side

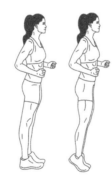

5 calf raises

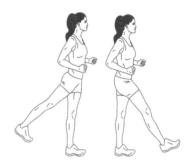

10 leg swings
right side

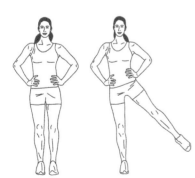

10 side leg raises
left side

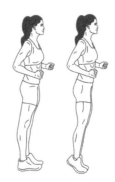

5 calf raises

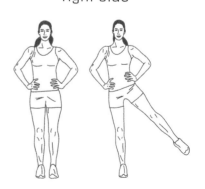

10 side leg raises
right side

#55

Best Self Workout

MY BEST SELF

WORKOUT
BY DAREBEE
© darebee.com

Level I 3 sets
Level II 5 sets
Level III 7 sets
2 minutes rest
in between

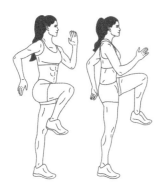

20 march steps

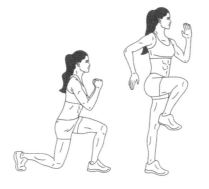

10 lunge step-ups

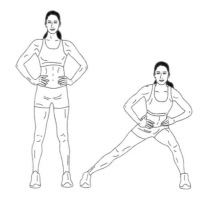

10 side lunges

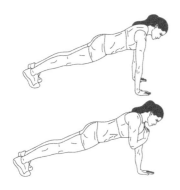

20 shoulder taps

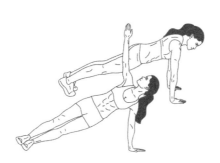

10 plank rotations

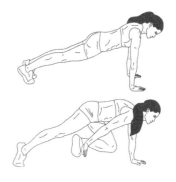

10 climber taps

#56

Blackbird Workout

Blackbird

DAREBEE WORKOUT © darebee.com

LEVEL I 3 sets **LEVEL II** 5 sets **LEVEL III** 7 sets **REST** up to 2 minutes

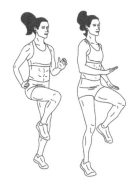

20 high knees

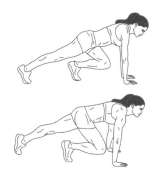

10 climbers

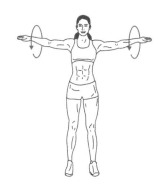

20 raised arm circles

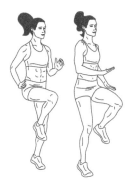

20 high knees

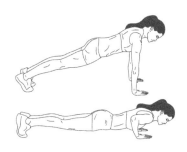

2 push-ups

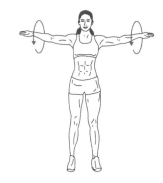

20 raised arm circles

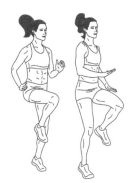

20 high knees

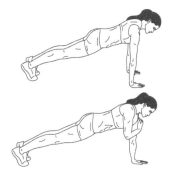

10 shoulder taps

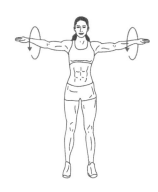

20 raised arm circles

#57

Burning Bright Workout

BURNING BRIGHT

DAREBEE WORKOUT © darebee.com

LEVEL I 3 sets **LEVEL II** 5 sets **LEVEL III** 7 sets **REST** up to 2 minutes

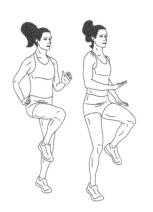

20 high knees

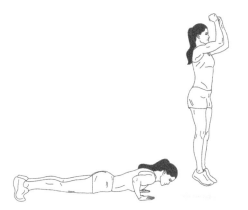

2 burpees

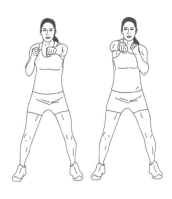

20 punches

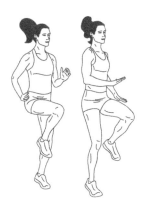

20 high knees

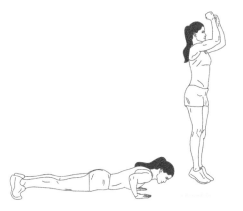

2 burpees

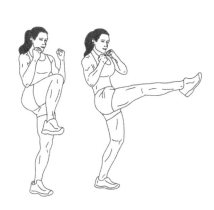

20 front kicks

#58

Burpee Queen Workout

BURPEE QUEEN

DAREBEE WORKOUT © **darebee.com**

Note: if you can't do push-ups,
do basic burpees instead.

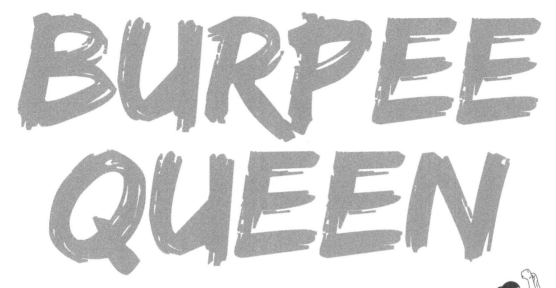

10 burpees

20-count rest

8 burpees

20-count rest

6 burpees

20-count rest

4 burpees

20-count rest

2 burpees

done

#59

Busy Bee Workout

Busy Bee

DAREBEE WORKOUT © darebee.com

LEVEL I 3 sets **LEVEL II** 5 sets **LEVEL III** 7 sets **REST** up to 2 minutes

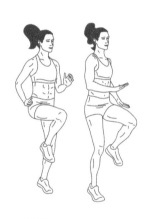

20 high knees

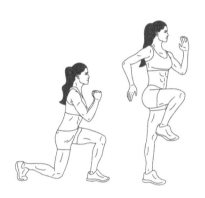

10 lunge step-ups

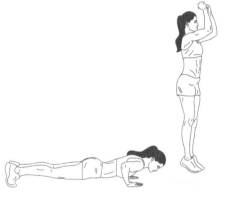

5 burpees

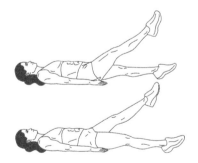

20 flutter kicks

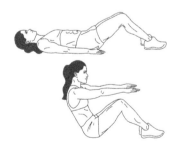

10 sit-ups

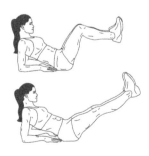

5 crunch kicks

#60

Cardio & Core Burn Workout

cardio & core burn

DAREBEE
WORKOUT
© darebee.com

Level I 3 sets
Level II 5 sets
Level III 7 sets
2 minutes rest between sets

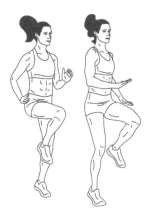

20 high knees

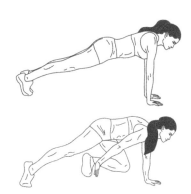

4 climber taps

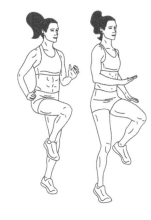

20 high knees

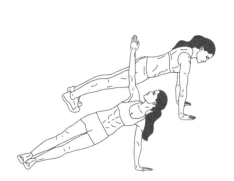

4 plank rotations

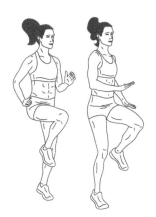

20 high knees

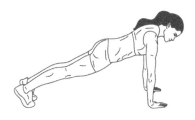

20-count plank hold

#61

Cardio & Core Express Workout

Cardio & Core

EXPRESS

DAREBEE
WORKOUT
© darebee.com
3 sets | 2 minutes rest

10 jumping jacks

4 knee-to-elbows

10 jumping jacks

4 knee-to-elbows

10 jumping jacks

4 knee-to-elbows

10 jumping jacks

4 knee-to-elbows

10 jumping jacks

4 knee-to-elbows

#62

Cardio Queen Workout

CARDIO QUEEN

DAREBEE WORKOUT © darebee.com

LEVEL I 3 sets **LEVEL II** 5 sets **LEVEL III** 7 sets **REST** up to 2 minutes

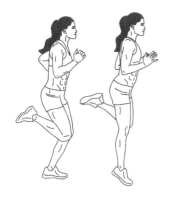

10 butt kicks

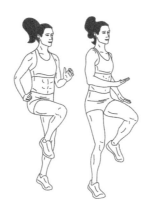

10 high knees

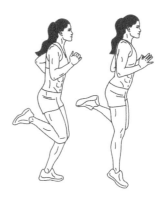

10 butt kicks

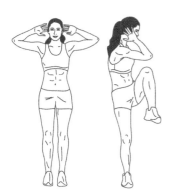

4 knee-to-elbows

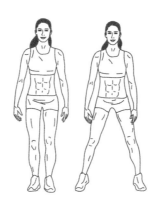

10 half jacks

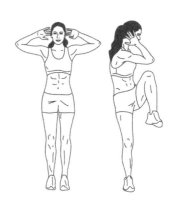

4 knee-to-elbows

#63

Caterpillar-Butterfly Workout

caterpillar-
Butterfly

DAREBEE WORKOUT © darebee.com

LEVEL I 3 sets **LEVEL II** 5 sets **LEVEL III** 7 sets **REST** up to 2 minutes

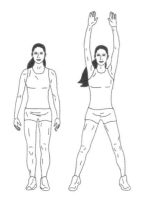

10 jumping jacks

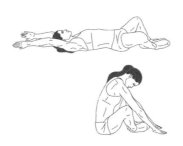

10 butterfly sit-ups

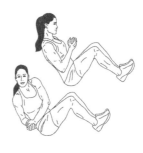

10 sitting twists

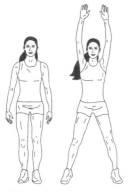

10 jumping jacks

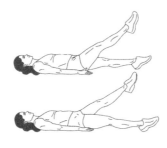

10 flutter kicks

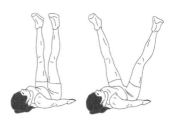

10 V-wipers

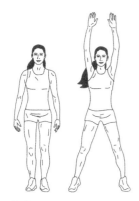

10 jumping jacks

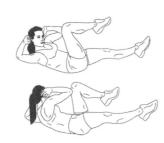

10 knee-to-elbow crunches

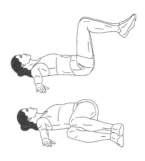

10 half wipers

#64

Chapter One Workout

Chapter 1

DAREBEE WORKOUT © darebee.com

LEVEL I 3 sets **LEVEL II** 5 sets **LEVEL III** 7 sets **REST** up to 2 minutes

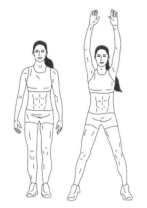
10 jumping jacks

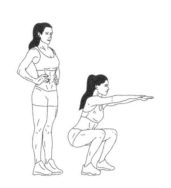
6 squats

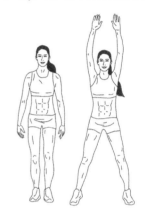
10 jumping jacks

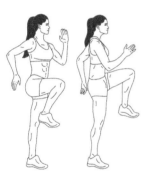
10 march steps

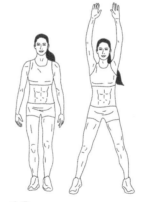
10 jumping jacks

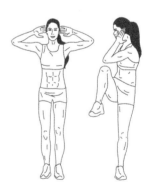
10 knee-to-elbow

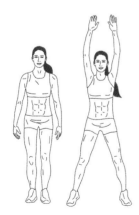
10 jumping jacks

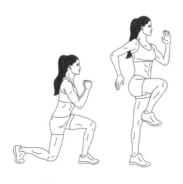
6 lunge step-up

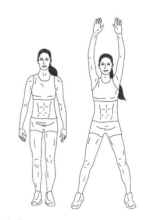
10 jumping jacks

#65

Cheeky Monkey Workout

Cheeky Monkey

DAREBEE WORKOUT
© darebee.com
Level I 3 sets
Level II 5 sets
Level III 7 sets
2 minutes rest

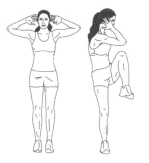

10 knee-to-elbows

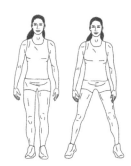

10 half jacks

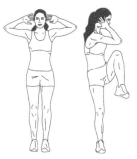

10 knee-to-elbows

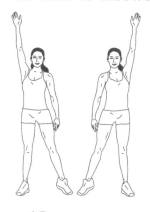

10 step jacks

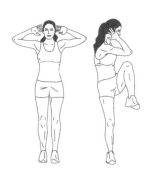

10 knee-to-elbows

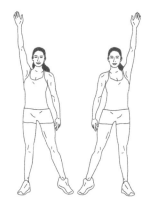

10 step jacks

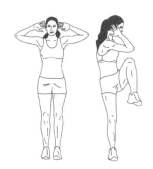

10 knee-to-elbows

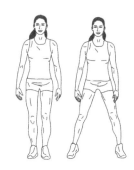

10 half jacks

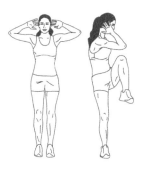

10 knee-to-elbows

#66

Cheetah Workout

CHEETAH

DAREBEE WORKOUT © darebee.com

LEVEL I 3 sets **LEVEL II** 5 sets **LEVEL III** 7 sets **REST** up to 2 minutes

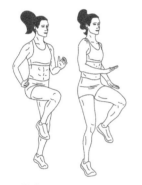

20 high knees

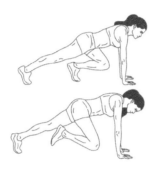

10 climbers

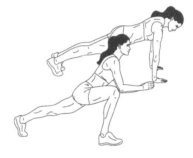

4 plank-into-lunges

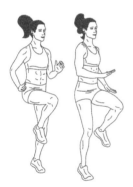

20 high knees

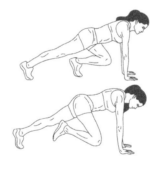

10 climbers

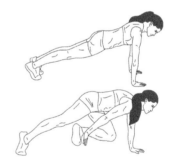

4 climber taps

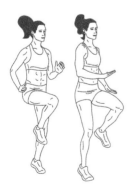

20 high knees

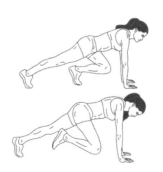

10 climbers

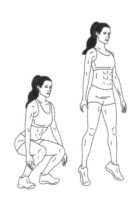

4 jump squats

#67

Clean Sweep Workout

CLEAN SWEEP

HIIT WORKOUT
BY DAREBEE
© darebee.com
Level I 3 sets
Level II 5 sets
Level III 7 sets
2 minutes rest

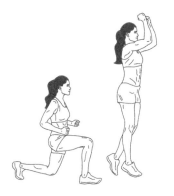

10sec jumping lunges

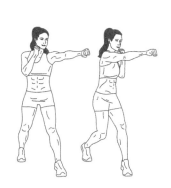

40sec punches

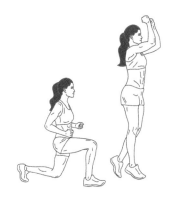

10sec jumping lunges

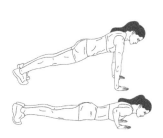

10sec push-ups

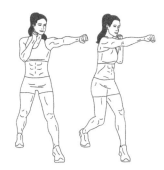

40sec punches

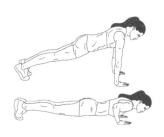

10sec push-ups

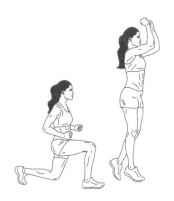

10sec jumping lunges

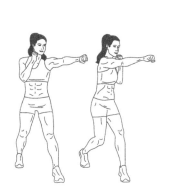

40sec punches

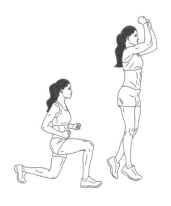

10sec jumping lunges

#68

Coda Workout

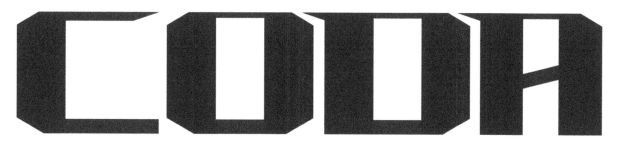

CODA

DAREBEE **HIIT** WORKOUT © darebee.com

Level I 3 sets **Level II** 5 sets **Level III** 7 sets

2 minutes rest between sets

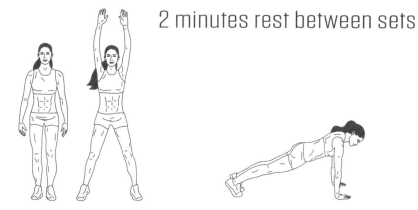

20sec jumping jacks

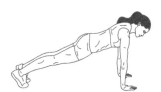

20sec plank hold

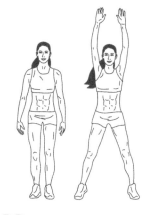

20sec jumping jacks

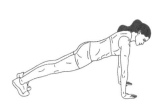

20sec plank hold

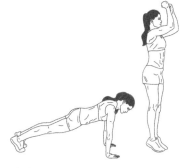

20sec basic burpees

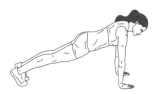

20sec plank hold

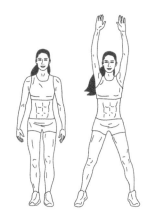

20sec jumping jacks

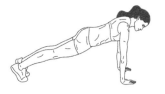

20sec plank hold

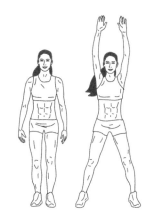

20sec jumping jacks

#69

Courage Workout

courage

DAREBEE WORKOUT © darebee.com

LEVEL I 3 sets **LEVEL II** 5 sets **LEVEL III** 7 sets **REST** up to 2 minutes

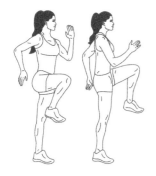

10 march steps

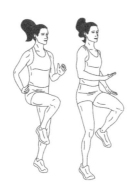

10 high knees

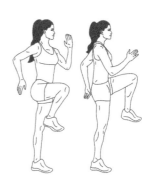

10 march steps

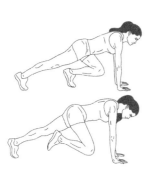

10 climbers

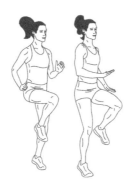

10 high knees

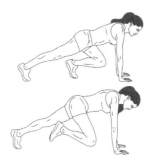

10 climbers

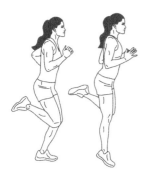

10 butt kicks

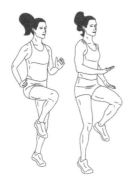

10 high knees

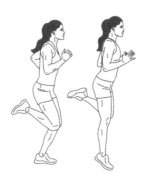

10 butt kicks

#70

Enigma Workout

ENIGMA

DAREBEE WORKOUT © darebee.com

LEVEL I 3 sets **LEVEL II** 5 sets **LEVEL III** 7 sets **REST** up to 2 minutes

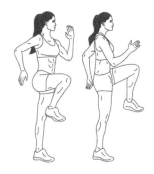

20 march steps

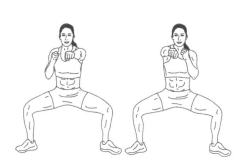

20 squat hold punches

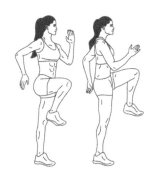

20 march steps

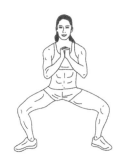

10-count squat hold

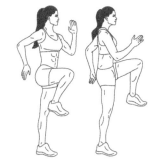

20 march steps

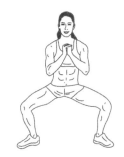

10-count squat hold

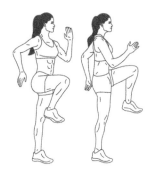

20 march steps

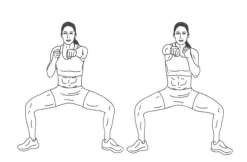

20 squat hold punches

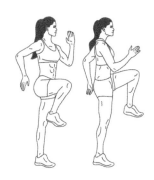

20 march steps

#71

Extra Spice Workout

EXTRA SPICE

DAREBEE WORKOUT
© darebee.com
Level I 3 sets
Level II 5 sets
Level III 7 sets
2 minutes rest

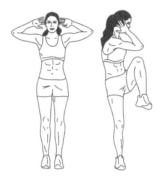

10 jumping jacks

10 knee-to-elbows

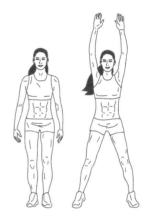

10 jumping jacks

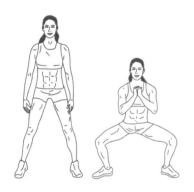

10 goblet squats

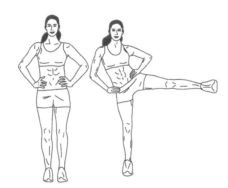

10 side leg raises

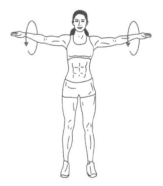

10 raised arm circles

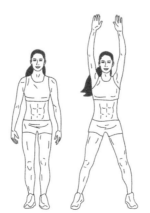

10 jumping jacks

#72

Fast & Dangerous Workout

Fast & Dangerous

DAREBEE HIIT WORKOUT © darebee.com

Level I 3 sets **Level II** 5 sets **Level III** 7 sets | 2 minutes rest

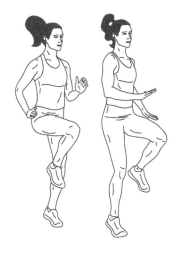

15sec high knees

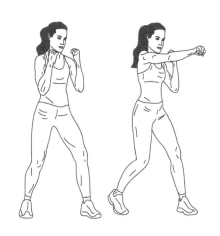

15sec punches

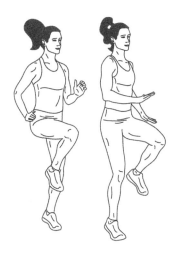

15sec high knees

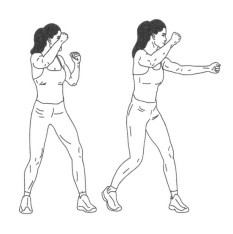

15sec backfists

#73

Feel Good Workout

feelgood

DAREBEE WORKOUT © darebee.com

LEVEL I 3 sets **LEVEL II** 4 sets **LEVEL III** 5 sets **REST** up to 2 minutes

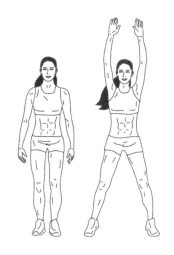

10 jumping jacks

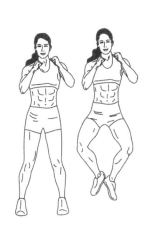

2 hop heel clicks

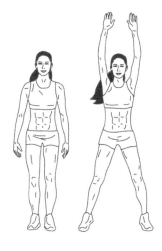

10 jumping jacks

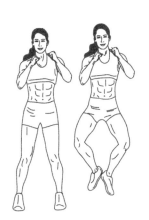

2 hop heel clicks

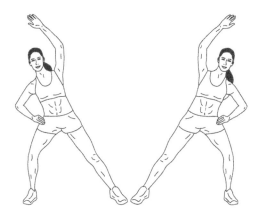

10 side jacks

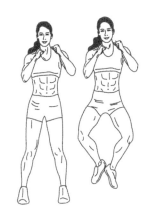

2 hop heel clicks

#74

Feral Workout

FERAL

DAREBEE WORKOUT © darebee.com

LEVEL I 3 sets **LEVEL II** 5 sets **LEVEL III** 7 sets **REST** up to 2 minutes

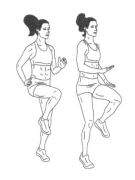

20 high knees

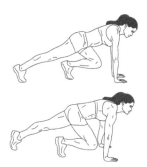

10 climbers

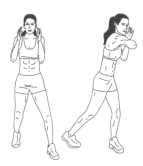

20 elbow strikes

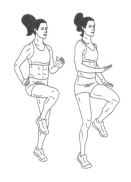

20 high knees

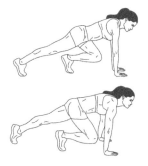

10 climbers

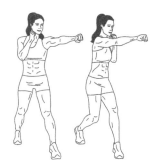

20 punches

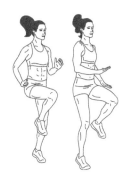

20 high knees

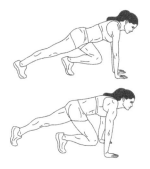

10 climbers

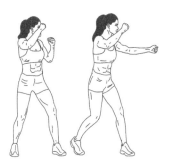

20 backfists

#75

Fire & Sweat Workout

Fire and Sweat

DAREBEE HIIT WORKOUT © darebee.com

Level I 3 sets **Level II** 5 sets **Level III** 7 sets | 2 minutes rest

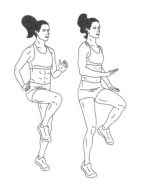

30sec high knees

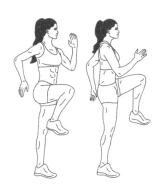

30sec march steps

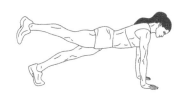

30sec raised leg plank hold

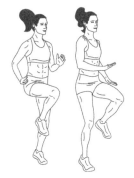

30sec high knees

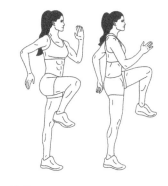

30sec march steps

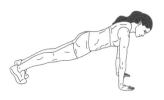

30sec plank hold

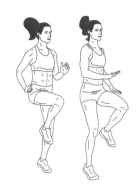

30sec high knees

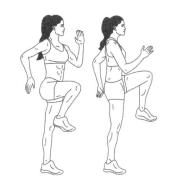

30sec march steps

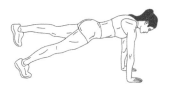

30sec raised leg plank hold

#76

Girl On Fire Workout

A GIRL ON FIRE

DAREBEE WORKOUT © darebee.com

LEVEL I 3 sets **LEVEL II** 5 sets **LEVEL III** 7 sets **REST** up to 2 minutes

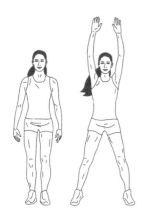

10 jumping jacks

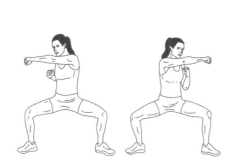

30 squat hold punches

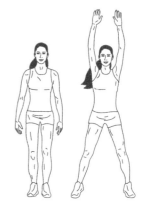

10 jumping jacks

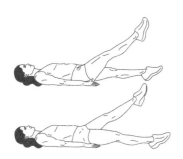

10 flutter kicks

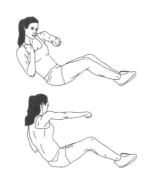

30 sitting punches

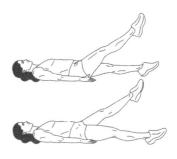

10 flutter kicks

#77

Glory Workout

GLORY

DAREBEE WORKOUT © darebee.com

LEVEL I 3 sets **LEVEL II** 5 sets **LEVEL III** 7 sets **REST** up to 2 minutes

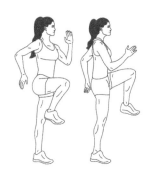

20 march steps

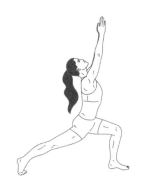

10-count hold

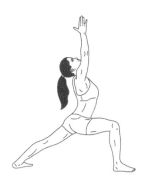

10-count hold

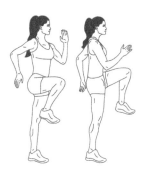

20 march steps

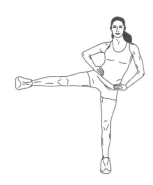

10-count balance hold

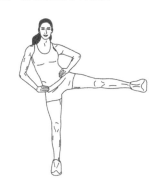

10-count balance hold

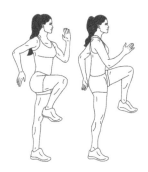

20 march steps

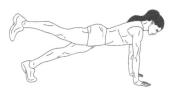

10-count plank hold

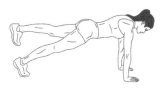

10-count plank hold

#78

Graceling Workout

Graceling

DAREBEE **HIIT** WORKOUT © darebee.com

Level I 3 sets **Level II** 5 sets **Level III** 7 sets | 2 minutes rest

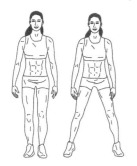

20sec half jacks

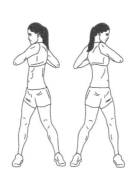

20sec twists

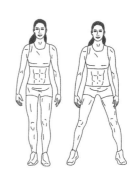

20sec half jacks

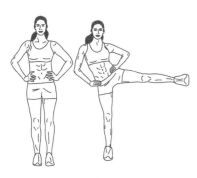

20sec side leg raises

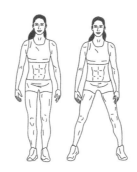

20sec half jacks

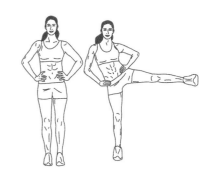

20sec side leg raises

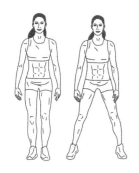

20sec half jacks

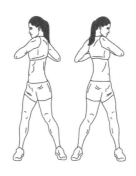

20sec twists

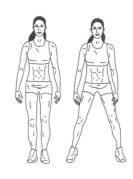

20sec half jacks

#79

Grit & Grace Workout

GRIT & GRACE

WORKOUT
BY DAREBEE
© darebee.com

Level I 3 sets
Level II 5 sets
Level III 7 sets
2 minutes rest

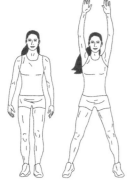

10 jumping jacks

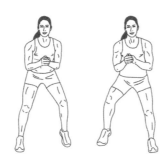

10 pacer steps

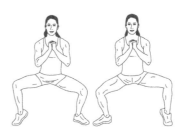

10 squat hold calf raises

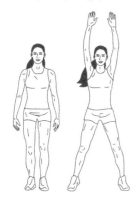

10 jumping jacks

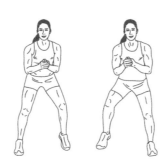

10 pacer steps

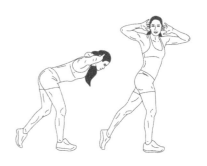

10 deadlifts with twist

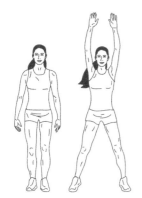

10 jumping jacks

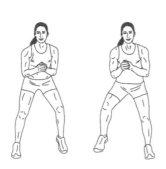

10 pacer steps

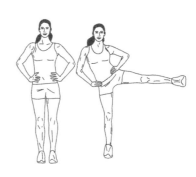

10 side leg raises

#80

Harbinger Workout

HARBINGER

DAREBEE WORKOUT © darebee.com

LEVEL I 3 sets **LEVEL II** 5 sets **LEVEL III** 7 sets **REST** up to 2 minutes

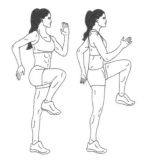
10 march steps

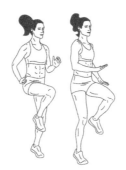
10 high knees

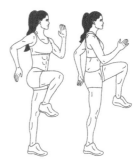
10 march steps

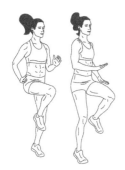
10 high knees

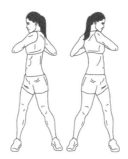
10 torso twists

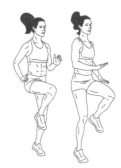
10 high knees

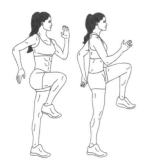
10 march steps

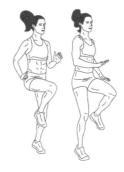
10 high knees

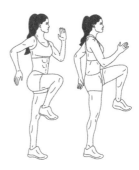
10 march steps

#81

Haywire Workout

Haywire

DAREBEE WORKOUT © darebee.com

LEVEL I 3 sets **LEVEL II** 5 sets **LEVEL III** 7 sets **REST** up to 2 minutes

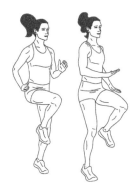

10 high knees

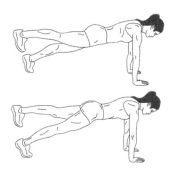

4 plank leg raises

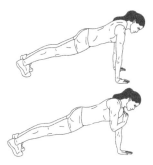

4 shoulder taps

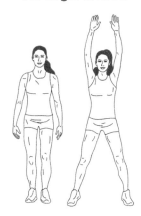

10 jumping jacks

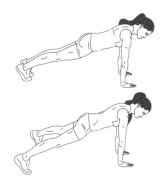

4 plank jacks

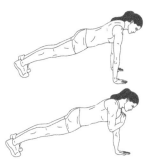

4 shoulder taps

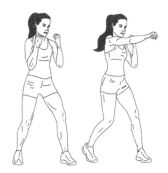

10 punches

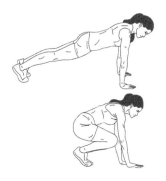

4 plank jump-ins

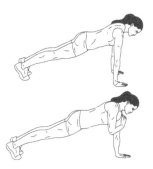

4 shoulder taps

#82

Hear Me Roar Workout

Hear Me Roar

DAREBEE **HIIT** WORKOUT © darebee.com

Level I 3 rounds **Level II** 5 rounds **Level III** 7 rounds 2 min rest between rounds

Extra Credit 1 push-up every 20 seconds

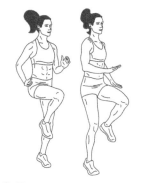

20sec high knees

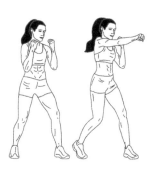

20sec punches

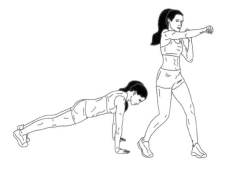

20sec plank + jab + cross

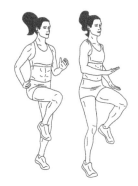

20sec high knees

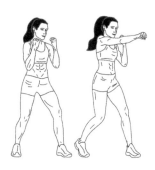

20sec punches

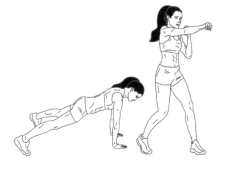

20sec plank jack + jab + cross

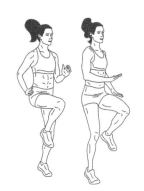

20sec high knees

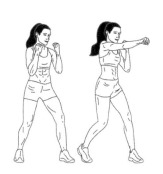

20sec punches

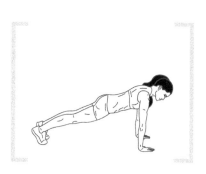

finish 20sec plank

#83

Hellion Workout

HELLION

DAREBEE WORKOUT © darebee.com

LEVEL I 3 sets **LEVEL II** 5 sets **LEVEL III** 7 sets **REST** up to 2 minutes

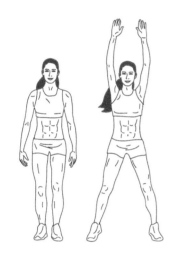

20 jumping jacks

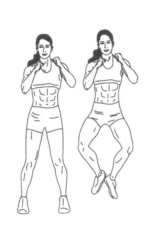

4 hop heel clicks

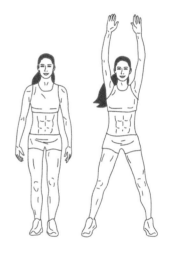

20 jumping jacks

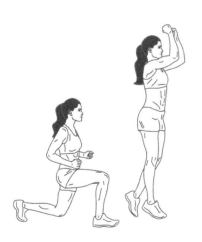

4 jumping lunges

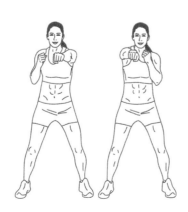

20 punches

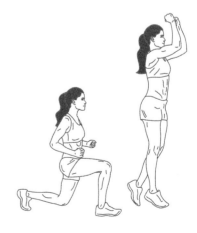

4 jumping lunges

#84

Kitsune Workout

kitsune

DAREBEE WORKOUT © darebee.com

LEVEL I 3 sets **LEVEL II** 5 sets **LEVEL III** 7 sets **REST** up to 2 minutes

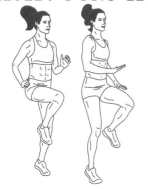

20 high knees

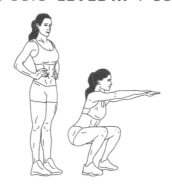

20 squats

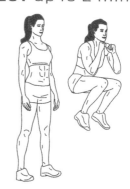

4 jump knee tucks

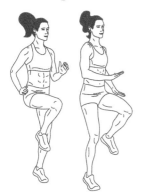

20 high knees

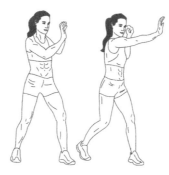

20 palm strikes

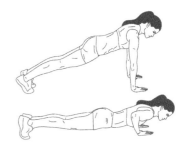

4 push-ups

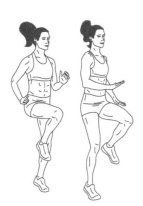

20 high knees

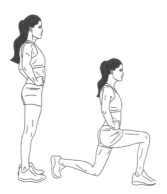

20 lunges

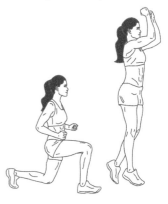

4 jumping lunges

#85

Lioness Workout

Lioness

LEVEL I 3 sets **LEVEL II** 5 sets **LEVEL III** 7 sets **REST** up to 2 minutes

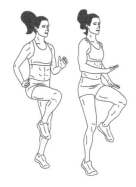

10 high knees

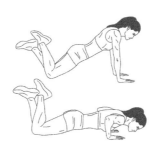

5 knee push-ups

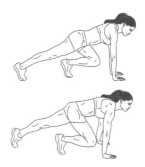

10 climbers

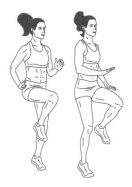

10 high knees

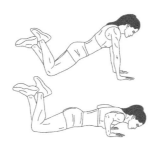

5 knee push-ups

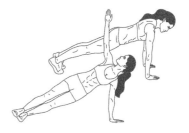

10 plank rotations

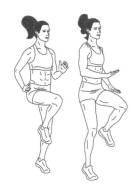

10 high knees

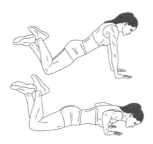

5 knee push-ups

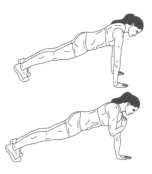

10 shoulder taps

#86

Mermaid Workout

MERMAID

DAREBEE WORKOUT © darebee.com

LEVEL I 3 sets **LEVEL II** 5 sets **LEVEL III** 7 sets **REST** up to 2 minutes

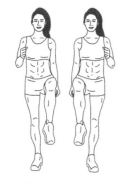

20 march steps

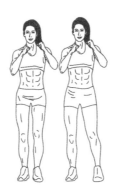

20 side steps

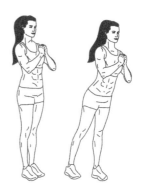

20 back steps

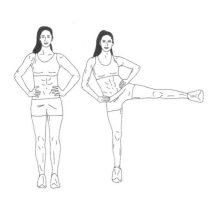

20 side leg raises

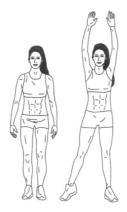

20 step jacks

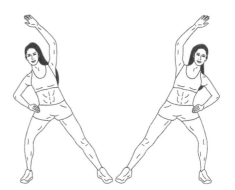

20 step side jacks

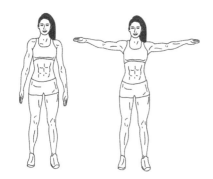

10 arm raises

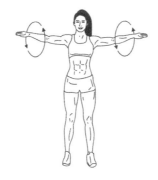

10 raised arm circles

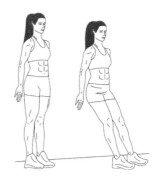

10 wall squats

#87

One Brave Girl Workout

ONE BRAVE GIRL

DAREBEE WORKOUT © darebee.com

LEVEL I 3 sets **LEVEL II** 5 sets **LEVEL III** 7 sets **REST** up to 2 minutes

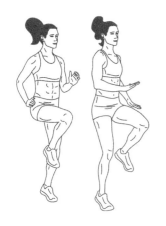

20 high knees

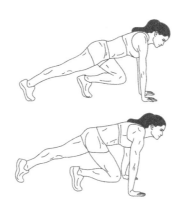

10 climbers

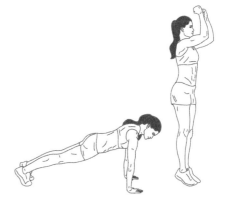

2 basic burpees

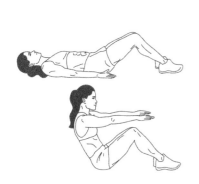

10 sit-ups

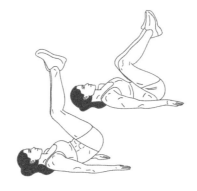

10 reverse crunches

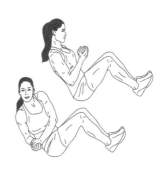

10 sitting twists

#88

Persephone Workout

PERSEPHONE

DAREBEE `HIIT` WORKOUT © darebee.com

Level I 3 sets **Level II** 5 sets **Level III** 7 sets | 2 minutes rest

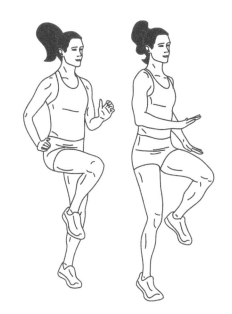

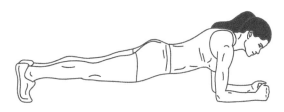

30sec high knees

30sec elbow plank

30sec high knees

30sec elbow plank

30sec high knees

30sec elbow plank

30sec high knees

30sec elbow plank

#89

Phantom Workout

PHANTOM

DAREBEE WORKOUT © darebee.com

LEVEL I 3 sets **LEVEL II** 5 sets **LEVEL III** 7 sets **REST** up to 2 minutes

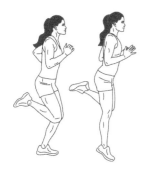

20 butt kicks

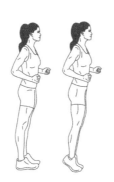

5 calf raises

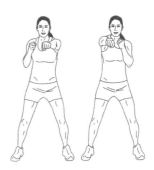

20 punches

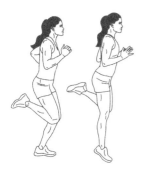

20 butt kicks

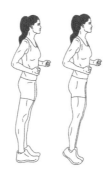

5 calf raises

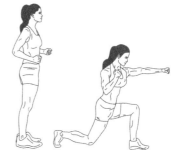

10 lunge punches

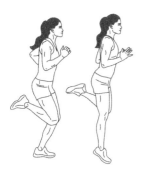

20 butt kicks

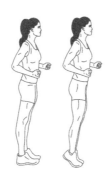

5 calf raises

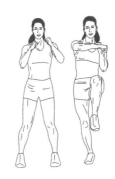

20 march hooks

#90

Rascal Workout

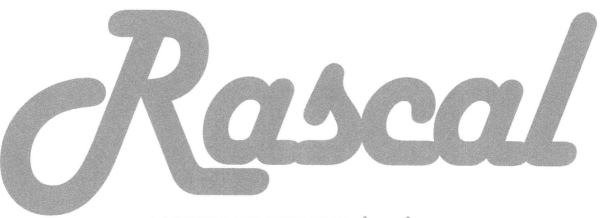

Rascal

DAREBEE WORKOUT © darebee.com
5 sets | 2 minutes rest between sets

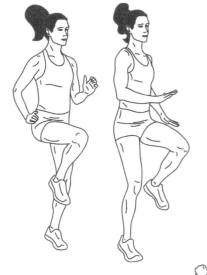

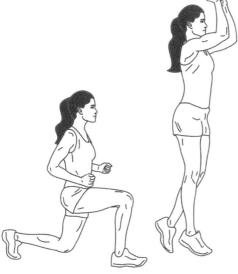

10 high knees

2 jumping lunges

10 high knees

2 jumping lunges

10 high knees

2 jumping lunges

10 high knees

2 jumping lunges

10 high knees

2 jumping lunges

#91

Raven Workout

RAVEN

DAREBEE WORKOUT © darebee.com

LEVEL I 3 sets **LEVEL II** 5 sets **LEVEL III** 7 sets **REST** up to 2 minutes

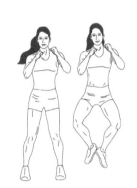

4 hop heel clicks

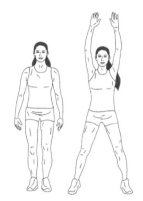

20 jumping jacks

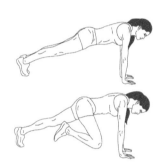

4 climbers

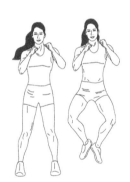

4 hop heel clicks

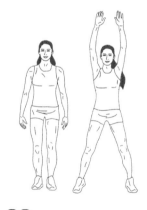

20 jumping jacks

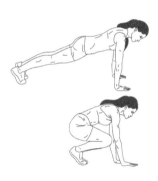

4 plank jump-ins

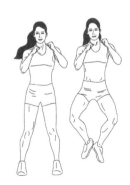

4 hop heel clicks

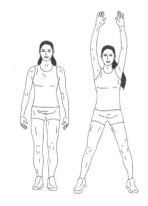

20 jumping jacks

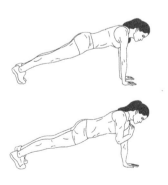

4 shoulder taps

#92

Ready Steady Go Workout

READY STEADY GO!

DAREBEE WORKOUT © darebee.com
LEVEL I 3 sets LEVEL II 4 sets LEVEL III 5 sets
REST up to 2 minutes

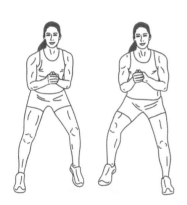

20 pacer steps

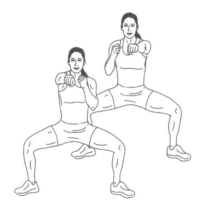

10 squat hold punches

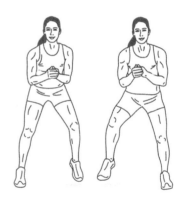

20 pacer steps

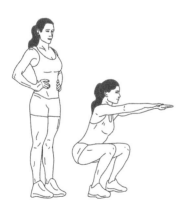

10 squats

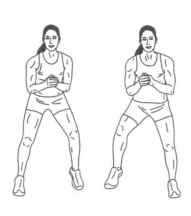

20 pacer steps

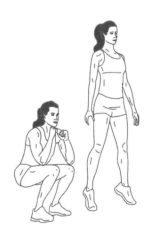

10 jump squats

#93

Shadow Workout

SHADOW

DAREBEE WORKOUT © darebee.com

LEVEL I 3 sets **LEVEL II** 5 sets **LEVEL III** 7 sets **REST** up to 2 minutes

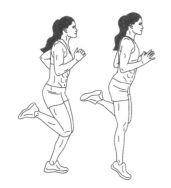

20 butt kicks

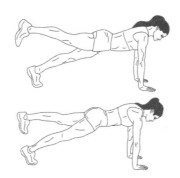

4 plank leg raises

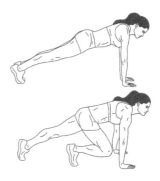

4 slow climbers

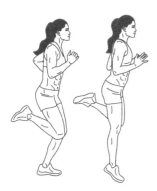

20 butt kicks

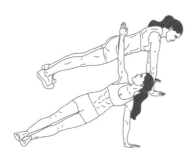

4 plank rotations

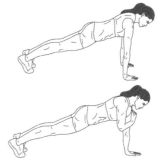

4 shoulder taps

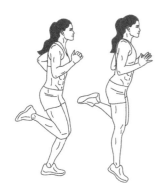

20 butt kicks

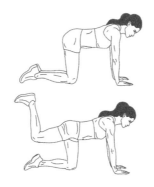

4 leg extensions

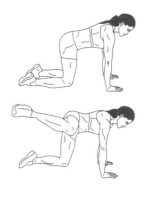

4 side leg extensions

#94

Siren Workout

SIREN

DAREBEE WORKOUT © darebee.com

LEVEL I 3 sets **LEVEL II** 5 sets **LEVEL III** 7 sets **REST** up to 2 minutes

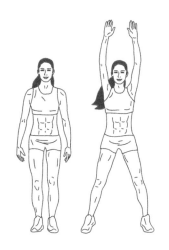

20 jumping jacks

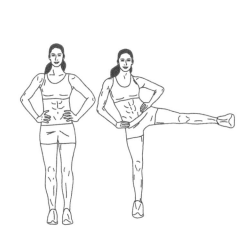

20 side leg raises

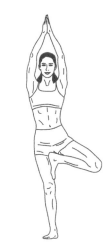

20-count balance hold

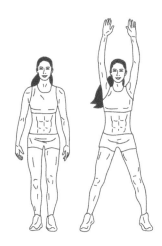

20 jumping jacks

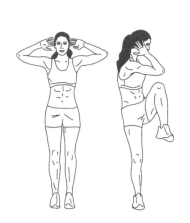

20 knee-to-elbows

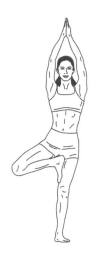

20-count balance hold

#95

Spright Workout

SPRIGHT

DAREBEE WORKOUT © darebee.com

LEVEL I 3 sets **LEVEL II** 5 sets **LEVEL III** 7 sets **REST** up to 2 minutes

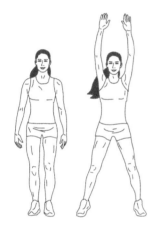

20 jumping jacks

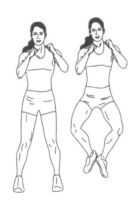

2 hop heel clicks

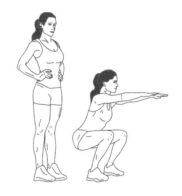

2 squats

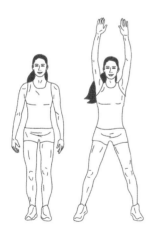

20 jumping jacks

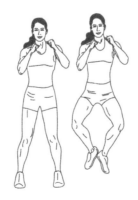

2 hop heel clicks

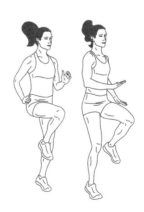

20 high knees

#96

Thunderbolt Workout

thunderbolt

DAREBEE `HIIT` WORKOUT © darebee.com

Level I 3 sets **Level II** 5 sets **Level III** 7 sets | 2 minutes rest

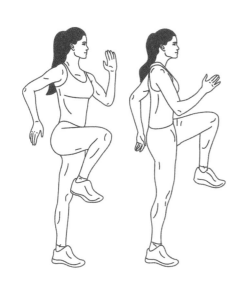 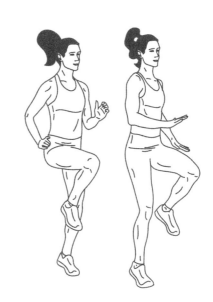

10sec march steps

10sec high knees

10sec march steps

10sec high knees

10sec march steps

10sec high knees

#97

What Doesnt Kill You Workout

What doesn't Kill you

DAREBEE WORKOUT
© darebee.com
Level I   3 sets
Level II 5 sets
Level III 7 sets
2 minutes rest

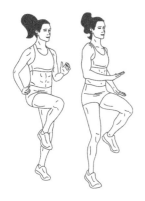

20 high knees

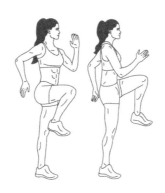

20 march steps

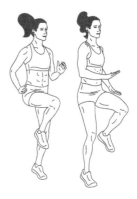

20 high knees

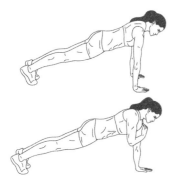

20 shoulder taps

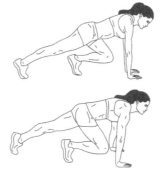

20 climbers

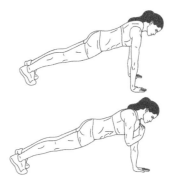

20 shoulder taps

#98

White Rabbit Workout

white rabbit

DAREBEE WORKOUT © darebee.com
5 sets in total | 2 minutes rest between sets

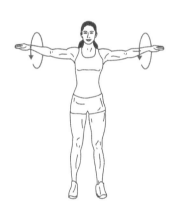 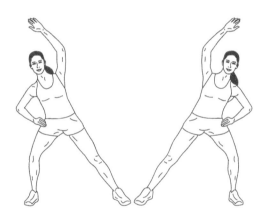 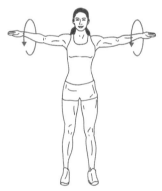

20 raised arm circles   **20** side jacks   **20** raised arm circles

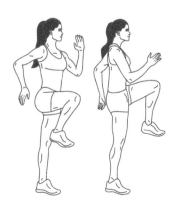 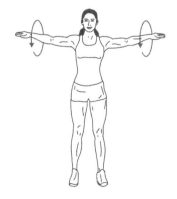 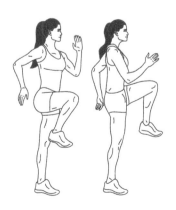

20 march steps   **20** raised arm circles   **20** march steps

#99

Wildfire Workout

WILDFIRE

LEVEL I 3 sets **LEVEL II** 5 sets **LEVEL III** 7 sets **REST** up to 2 minutes

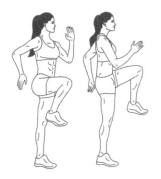

20 march steps

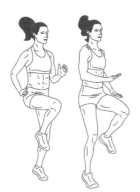

20 high knees

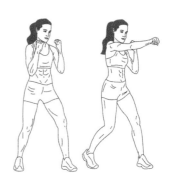

20 punches

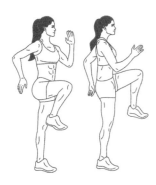

20 march steps

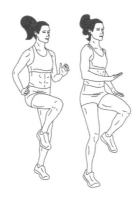

20 high knees

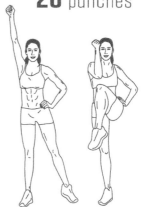

20 knee-to-elbow

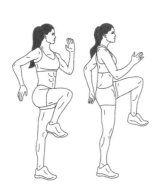

20 march steps

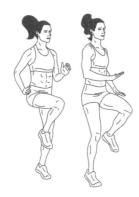

20 high knees

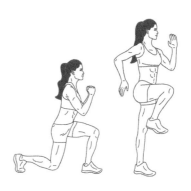

20 lunge step-ups

#100

That Workout I Promised

THAT WORKOUT
I PROMISED

DAREBEE WORKOUT © darebee.com

LEVEL I 3 sets **LEVEL II** 5 sets **LEVEL III** 7 sets **REST** up to 2 minutes

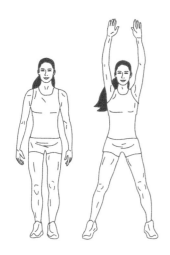

20 jumping jacks

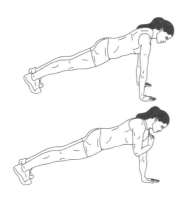

20 shoulder taps

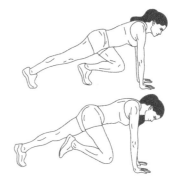

20 climbers

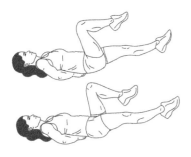

10 bicycle crunches

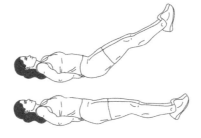

10 leg raises

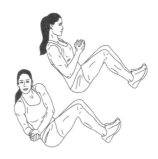

10 sitting twists

#101

Battle Angel Workout

Battle Angel

DAREBEE WORKOUT © darebee.com

LEVEL I 3 sets **LEVEL II** 5 sets **LEVEL III** 7 sets **REST** up to 2 minutes

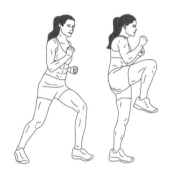

20 knee strikes

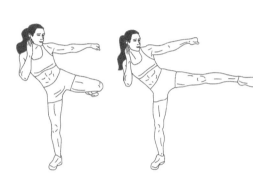

20 turning kicks

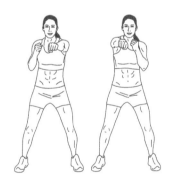

20 punches

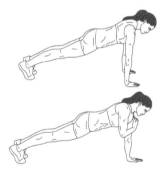

4 shoulder taps

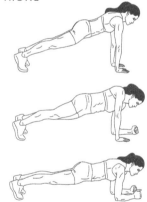

4 up and down planks

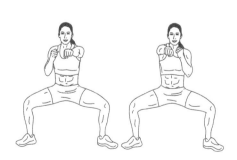

20 squat hold punches

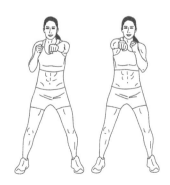

20 punches

#102

Brave New Me Workout

BRAVE NEW ME

DAREBEE WORKOUT © darebee.com

LEVEL I 3 sets **LEVEL II** 5 sets **LEVEL III** 7 sets **REST** up to 2 minutes

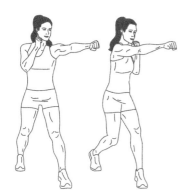

20 punches

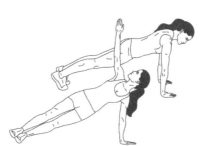

10 plank rotations

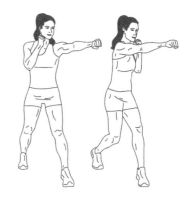

20 punches

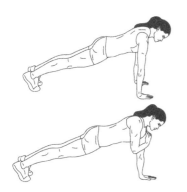

20 shoulder taps

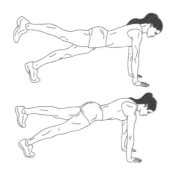

10 plank leg raises

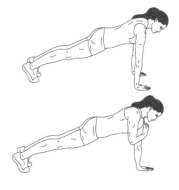

20 shoulder taps

#103

Brave Today Workout

I'M GOING TO BE
BRAVE TODAY

DAREBEE WORKOUT © darebee.com

LEVEL I 3 sets **LEVEL II** 5 sets **LEVEL III** 7 sets **REST** up to 2 minutes

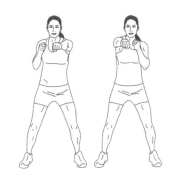

20 punches

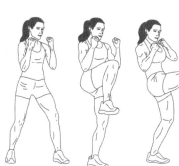

10 front kicks

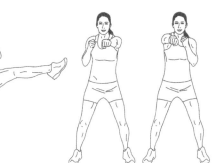

20 punches

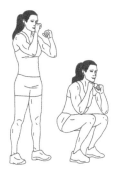

5 squats

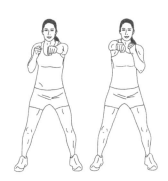

20 punches

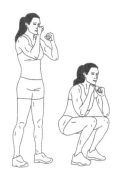

5 squats

#104

Captain Workout

CAPTAIN

DAREBEE HIIT WORKOUT © darebee.com

Level I 3 sets **Level II** 5 sets **Level III** 7 sets | 2 minutes rest

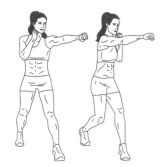

20sec punches

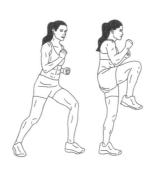

20sec knee strikes

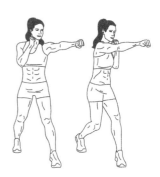

20sec punches

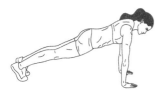

20sec plank hold

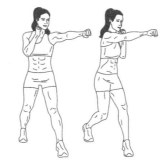

20sec punches

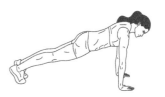

20sec plank hold

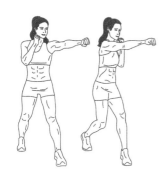

20sec punches

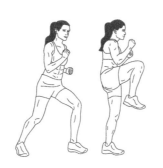

20sec knee strikes

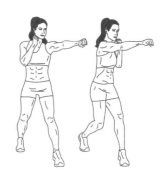

20sec punches

#105

Counter Workout

COUNTER

DAREBEE WORKOUT © darebee.com

LEVEL I 3 sets **LEVEL II** 5 sets **LEVEL III** 7 sets **REST** up to 2 minutes

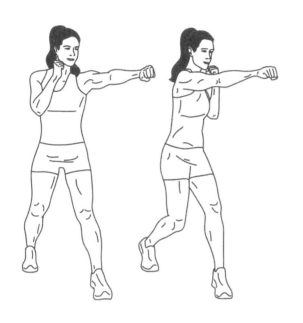

20 punches

2 squats

20 punches

2 squats

20 punches

2 squats

20 punches

2 squats

20 punches

2 squats

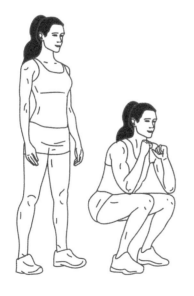

#106

Cyberpunk Workout

CYBERPUNK

DAREBEE WORKOUT © darebee.com

LEVEL I 3 sets **LEVEL II** 5 sets **LEVEL III** 7 sets **REST** up to 2 minutes

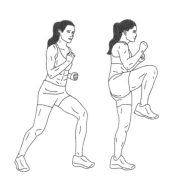

20 knee strikes

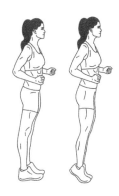

6 calf raises

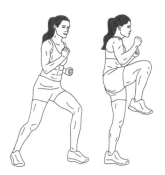

20 knee strikes

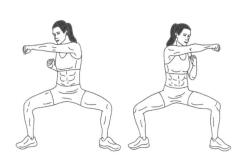

20 squat hold punches

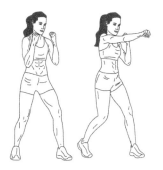

20 punches

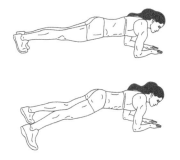

10 elbow plank step outs

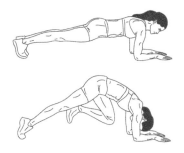

6 elbow plank knee-ins

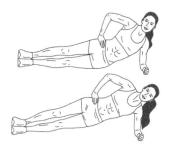

10 side bridges

#107

Dagger Workout

DAGGER

DAREBEE WORKOUT © darebee.com

LEVEL I 3 sets **LEVEL II** 5 sets **LEVEL III** 7 sets **REST** up to 2 minutes

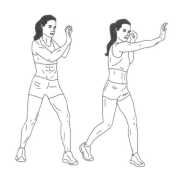

20 palm strikes

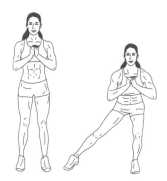

8 side lunges

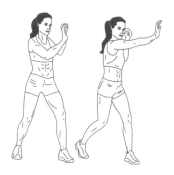

20 palm strikes

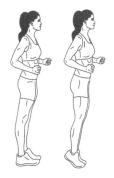

20 calf raises

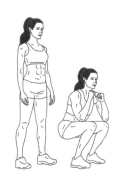

8 squats

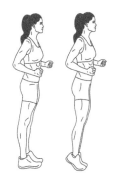

20 calf raises

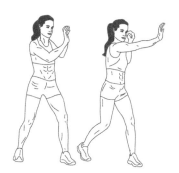

20 palm strikes

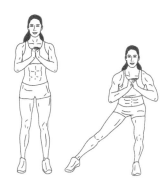

8 side lunges

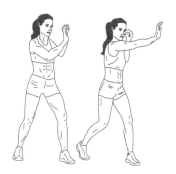

20 palm strikes

#108

Dryad Workout

DRYAD

DAREBEE WORKOUT © darebee.com

LEVEL I 3 sets **LEVEL II** 5 sets **LEVEL III** 7 sets **REST** up to 2 minutes

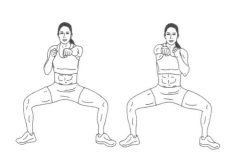

20 squat hold punches

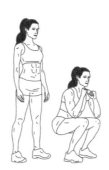

10 squats

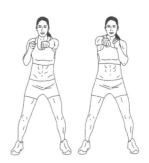

20 punches

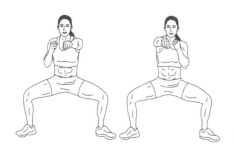

20 squat hold punches

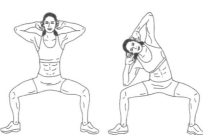

10 squat hold side bends

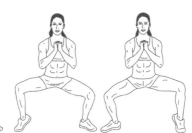

20 squat hold calf raises

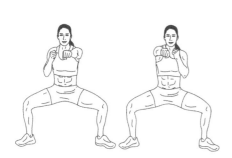

20 squat hold punches

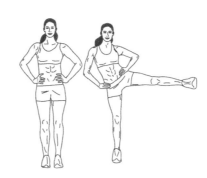

10 side leg raises

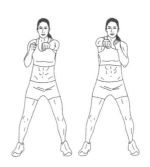

20 punches

#109

Fireheart Workout

FIREHEART

DAREBEE `HIIT` WORKOUT © darebee.com

Level I 3 sets **Level II** 5 sets **Level III** 7 sets | 2 minutes rest

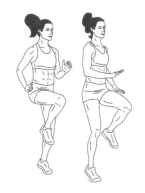

20sec high knees

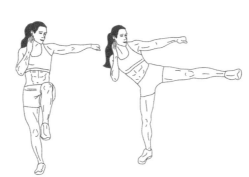

20sec side kicks

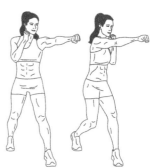

20sec punches

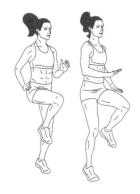

20sec high knees

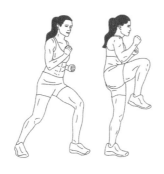

20sec knee strikes

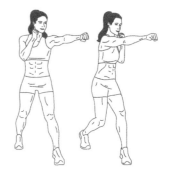

20sec punches

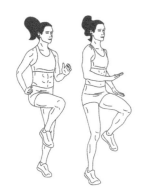

20sec high knees

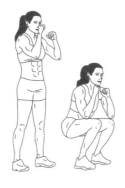

20sec squats

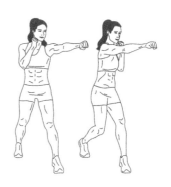

20sec punches

#110

Furyborn Workout

FURYBORN

DAREBEE WORKOUT © darebee.com

LEVEL I 3 sets **LEVEL II** 5 sets **LEVEL III** 7 sets **REST** up to 2 minutes

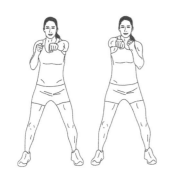

20 punches

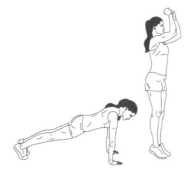

5 basic burpees

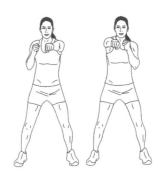

20 punches

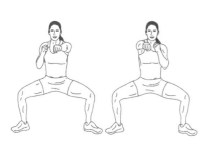

20 squat hold punches

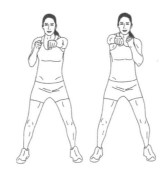

20 punches

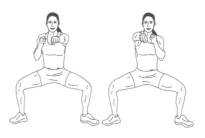

20 squat hold punches

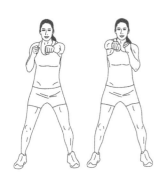

20 punches

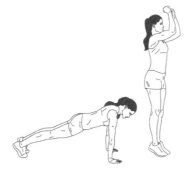

5 basic burpees

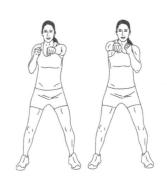

20 punches

#111

Mayhem Workout

MAYHEM

DAREBEE WORKOUT © darebee.com

LEVEL I 3 sets **LEVEL II** 5 sets **LEVEL III** 7 sets **REST** up to 2 minutes

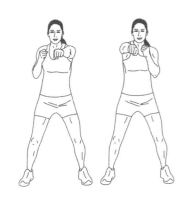

20 punches

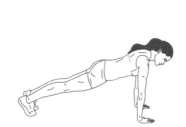

20-count plank hold

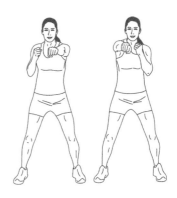

20 punches

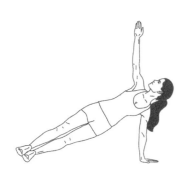

20-count side plank hold left side

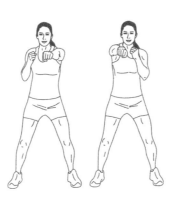

20 punches

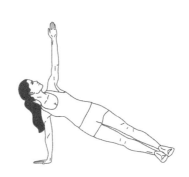

20-count side plank hold right side

#112

Maze Workout

MAZE

DAREBEE WORKOUT © darebee.com

LEVEL I 3 sets **LEVEL II** 5 sets **LEVEL III** 7 sets **REST** up to 2 minutes

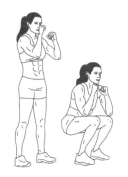

4 squats

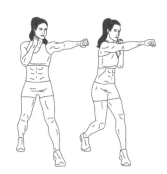

20 punches

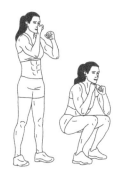

4 squats

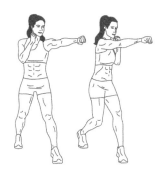

20 punches

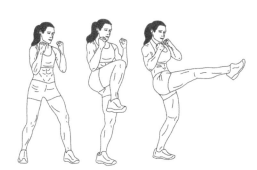

20 front kicks

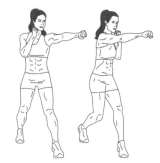

20 punches

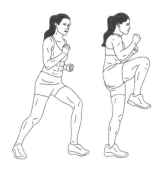

4 knee strikes

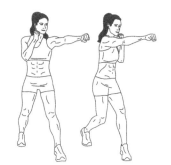

20 punches

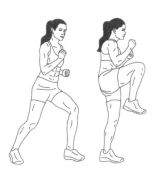

4 knee strikes

#113

Modern Girl Workout

MODERN GIRL

LEVEL I 3 sets **LEVEL II** 5 sets **LEVEL III** 7 sets **REST** up to 2 minutes

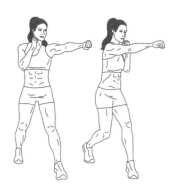

40 punches

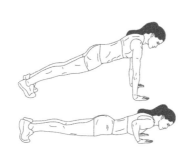

10 push-ups

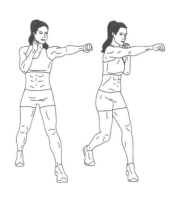

40 punches

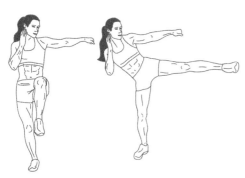

20 side kicks

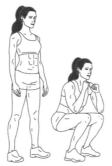

10 squats

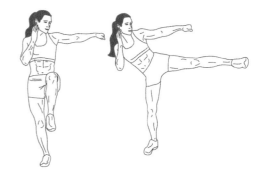

20 side kicks

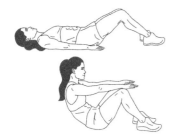

10 sit-ups

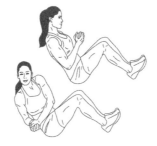

10 sitting twists

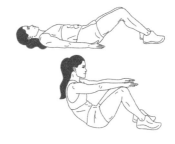

10 sit-ups

#114

Moxie Workout

MOXIE

DAREBEE WORKOUT © darebee.com

LEVEL I 3 sets **LEVEL II** 5 sets **LEVEL III** 7 sets **REST** up to 2 minutes

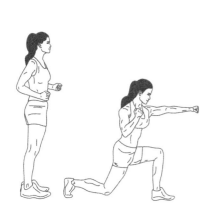

10 lunge punches

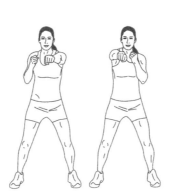

10 punches

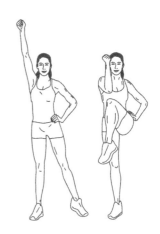

10 knee to elbows

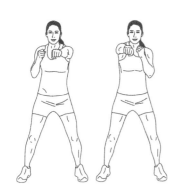

10 punches

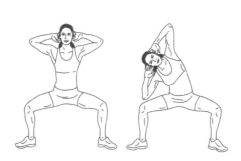

10 squat hold side bends

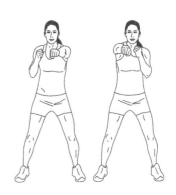

10 punches

#115

Ninja Princess Workout

ninja PRINCESS

DAREBEE WORKOUT © darebee.com

LEVEL I 3 sets **LEVEL II** 5 sets **LEVEL III** 7 sets **REST** up to 2 minutes

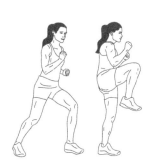

10 knee strikes

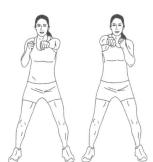

20 punches

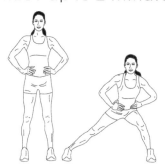

10 side lunges

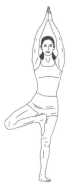

10-count tree pose hold

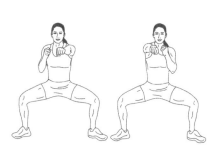

20 squat hold punches

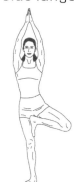

10-count tree pose hold

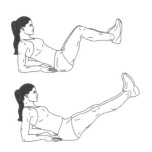

10 crunch kicks

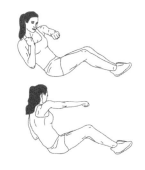

20 sitting punches

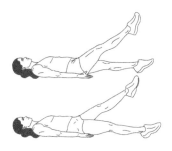

10 flutter kicks

#116

Onna Bugeisha Workout

ONNA BUGEISHA

DAREBEE WORKOUT © darebee.com

LEVEL I 3 sets **LEVEL II** 5 sets **LEVEL III** 7 sets **REST** up to 2 minutes

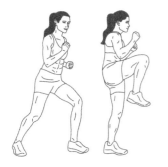

30 knee strikes

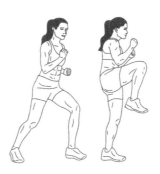

30combos knee strike + elbow strike

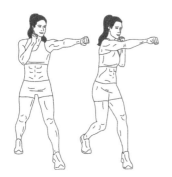

30 punches (jab + cross)

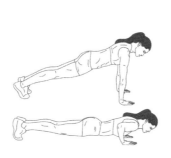

30combos push-up+ jab + cross

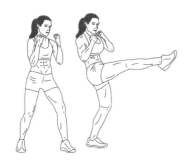

30 front kicks

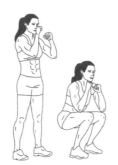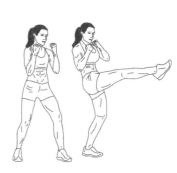

30combos squat + front kick

#117

Rage Workout

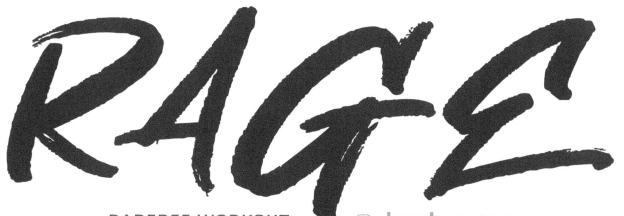

RAGE

DAREBEE WORKOUT © darebee.com

LEVEL I 3 sets **LEVEL II** 5 sets **LEVEL III** 7 sets **REST** up to 2 minutes

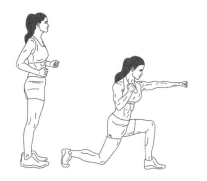

10 lunge punches

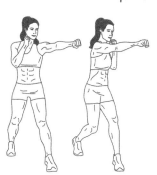

20 punches

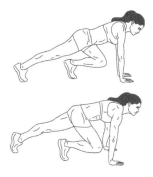

10 climbers

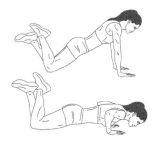

2 knee push-ups

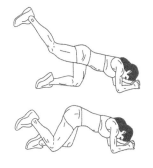

10 plank back kicks

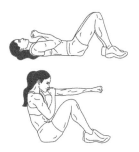

2 sit-up punches

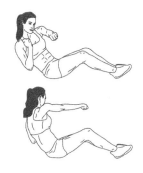

10 sitting punches

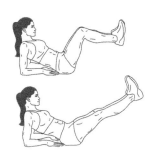

10 crunch kicks

#118

Shieldmaiden Workout

shieldmaiden

DAREBEE WORKOUT © darebee.com

LEVEL I 3 sets **LEVEL II** 5 sets **LEVEL III** 7 sets **REST** up to 2 minutes

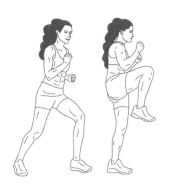

10 knee strikes

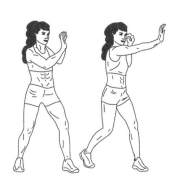

10 palm strikes

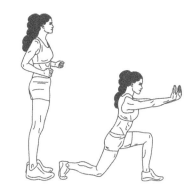

10 lunge push strikes

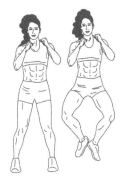
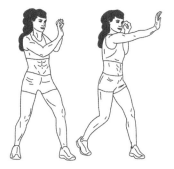

10combos hop heel click + palm strike

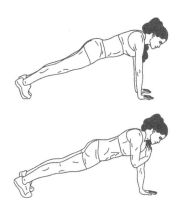

2 push-ups

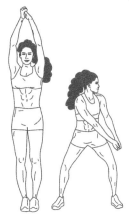

10 cross chops

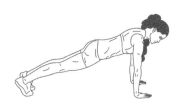

10-count plank hold

10 shoulder taps

#119

Warrior Queen Workout

WARRIOR QUEEN

DAREBEE WORKOUT © darebee.com

LEVEL I 3 sets **LEVEL II** 5 sets **LEVEL III** 7 sets **REST** up to 2 minutes

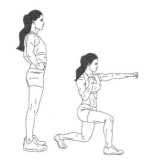

10 lunge punches

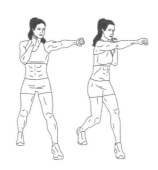

20 punches

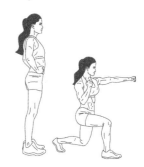

10 lunge punches

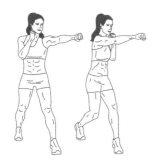

20 punches

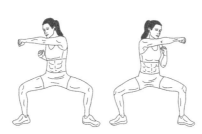

20 squat hold punches

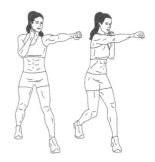

20 punches

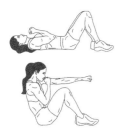

10 sit-up punches

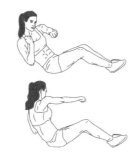

20 sitting punches

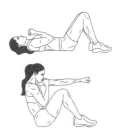

10 sit-up punches

#120

Wild & Free Workout

NOTES

WILD & FREE

DAREBEE WORKOUT
© darebee.com
LEVEL I   3 sets
LEVEL II   5 sets
LEVEL III 7 sets
REST up to 2 minutes

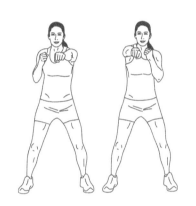

20 punches

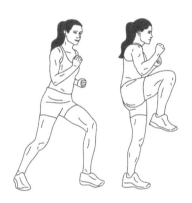

20 knee strikes

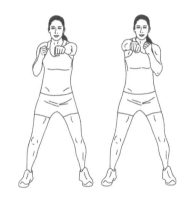

20 punches

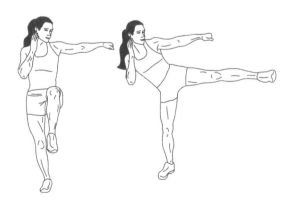

20 side kicks

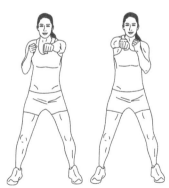

20 punches

#121

Backup & Restore Workout

Backup & Restore

DAREBEE WORKOUT
© darebee.com

slowly move
from one position
to the next;
hold each pose
for 4 seconds

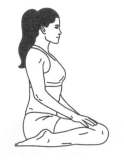

hero pose

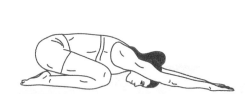

child's pose

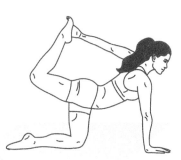

reach

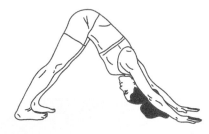

downward dog

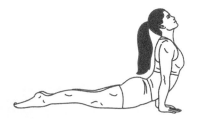

upward dog

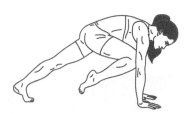

knee-in (each leg)

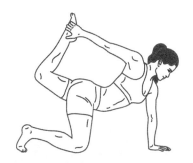

reach

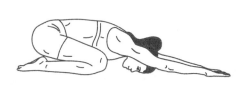

child's pose

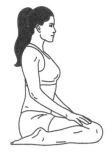

hero pose

#122

Better Balance Workout

Better Balance

DAREBEE WORKOUT © darebee.com
Change sides and repeat the sequence.

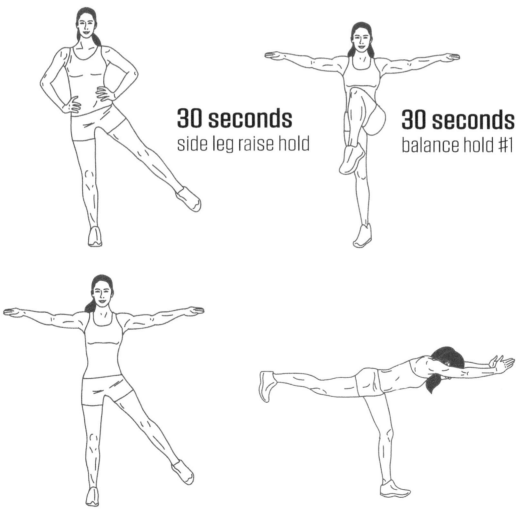

30 seconds side leg raise hold

30 seconds balance hold #1

30 seconds balance hold #2

30 seconds balance hold #3

#123

Better Sleep Yoga Workout

better
sleep

DAREBEE WORKOUT © darebee.com

Hold each pose for 20 seconds then move on to the next one.
Repeat each sequence again on the other side.

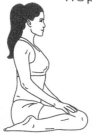 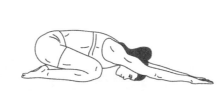 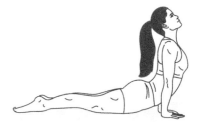

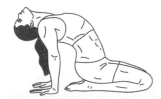 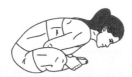 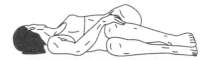

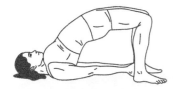 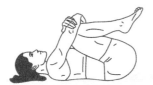 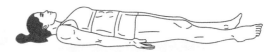

#124

Body Flow Workout

Body Flow

DAREBEE WORKOUT © darebee.com

Hold each pose for 20 seconds then move on to the next one.
Repeat the sequence again on the other side.

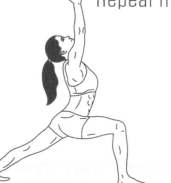

1. warrior I

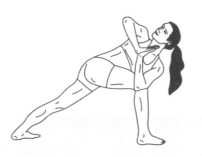

2. warrior side lotus

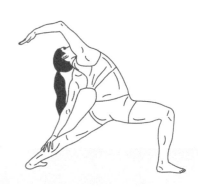

3. reverse warrior

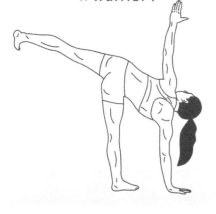

4. half moon

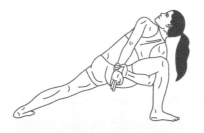

5. lunge lock

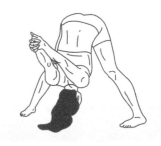

6. forward bend

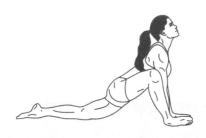

7. lizzard

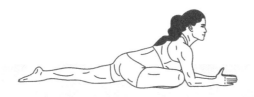

8. pigeon

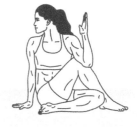

9. half lotus twist

#125

Centered Workout

Centered

DAREBEE WORKOUT © darebee.com

Hold each pose for 20 seconds then move on to the next one.
Repeat each sequence again on the other side.

SEQUENCE #1

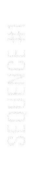 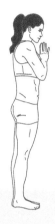 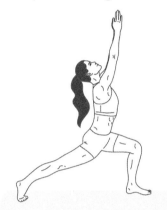 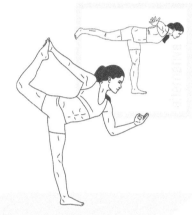

SEQUENCE #2

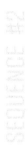 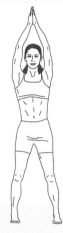 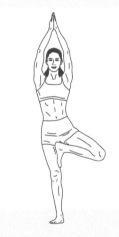 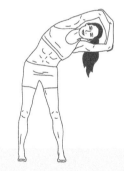

SEQUENCE #3

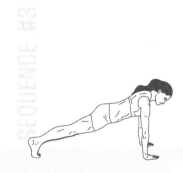 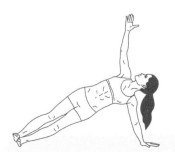 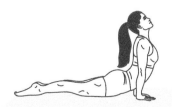

#126

De-Stress Yoga Fix Workout

DE-STRESS
YOGA FIX

by DAREBEE © darebee.com
Change sides and repeat.

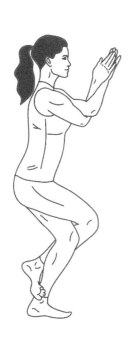 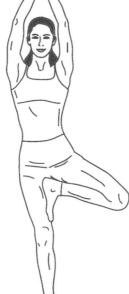 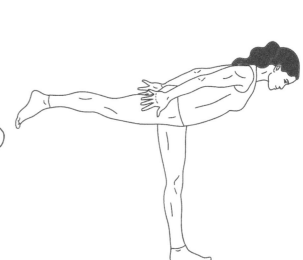

Eagle	Tree Pose	Warrior III
30 seconds	**30** seconds	**30** seconds

#127

Everyday Yoga Workout

EVERYDAY
YOGA

DAREBEE WORKOUT © darebee.com

Hold each pose for 20 seconds then move on to the next one.
Repeat the sequence again on the other side.

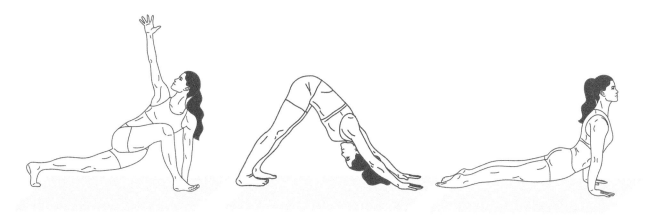

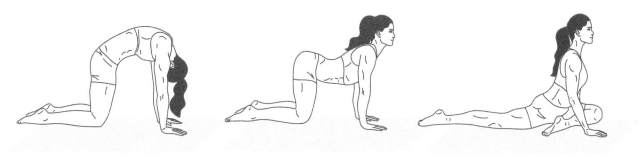

#128

Face The Day Workout

FACE the DAY

DAREBEE
WORKOUT
© darebee.com

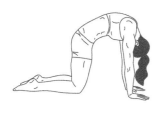
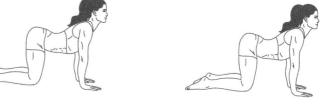

hold each pose for 20 seconds
change sides and repeat the sequence again

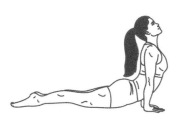

hold each for 5 seconds
repeat the sequence 5 times

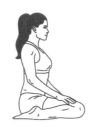

5 quick exhalations

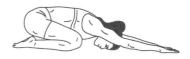

**hold the pose
for 20 seconds**

**hold the pose
for 20 seconds**

**hold the pose
for 60 seconds**

#129

Glow Workout

GLOW

DAREBEE WORKOUT © darebee.com

Hold each pose for 30 seconds then move on to the next one.
Repeat the sequence again on the other side.

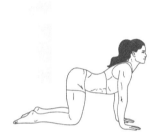 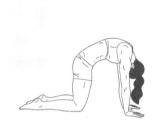 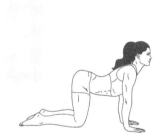

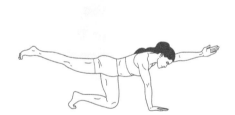 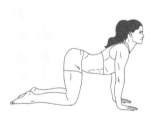 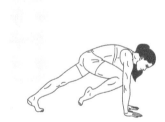

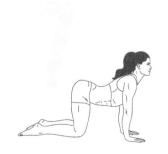 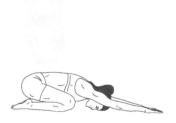 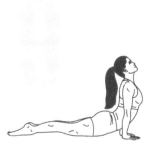

#130

Good Morning Yoga Workout

GOOD MORNING
YOGA

BY DAREBEE
Ⓒ darebee.com
Hold each pose
for **30 seconds**
then move on
to the next one.

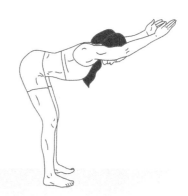

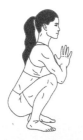
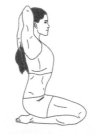
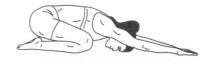

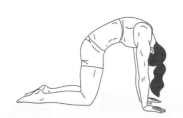
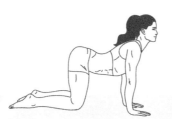
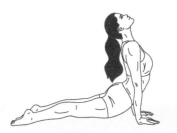

#131

Insomnia Yoga Workout

INSOMNIA
YOGA

DAREBEE WORKOUT © **darebee.com**

Hold each pose for 30 seconds then move on to the next one.

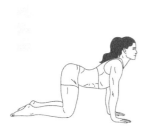
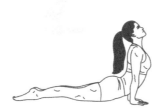
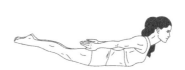

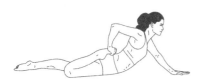
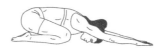
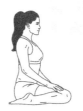

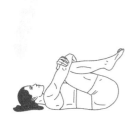
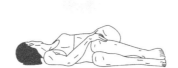
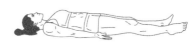

#132

Morning Ritual Workout

Morning Ritual

DAREBEE WORKOUT © darebee.com

Hold each pose for 30 seconds then move on to the next one.

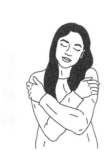 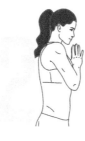 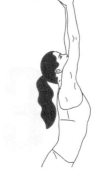

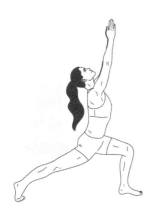 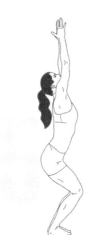 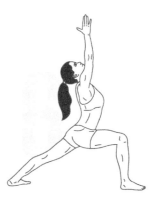

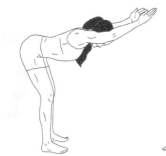 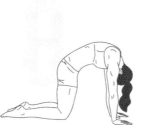 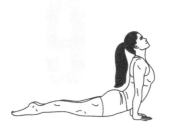

#133

Optimized Workout

OPTIMIZED

DAREBEE WORKOUT © darebee.com

Hold each pose for 30 seconds then move on to the next one.
Change sides and repeat the sequence.

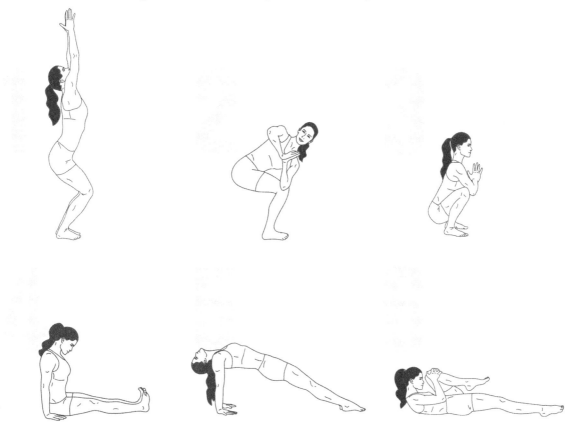

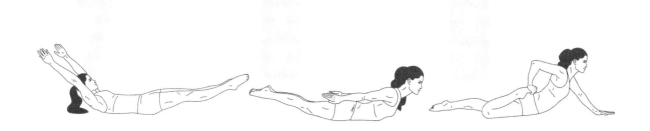

#134

Rawr Workout

rawr

DAREBEE WORKOUT © darebee.com

Hold each pose for 20 seconds then move on to the next one.
Repeat the sequence again on the other side.

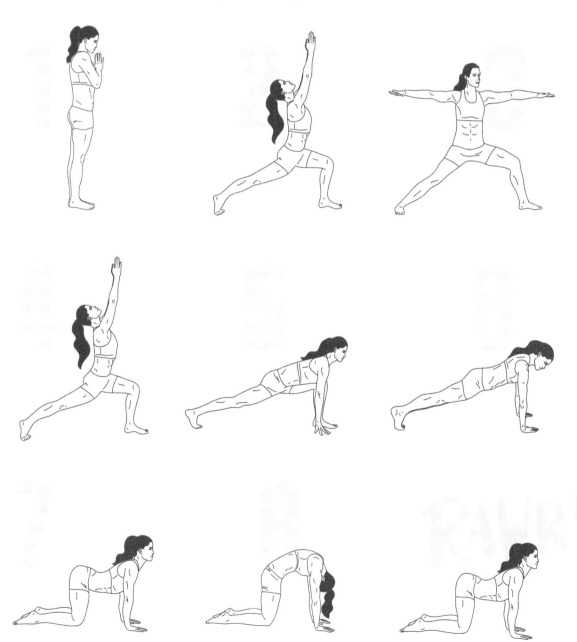

#135

Recovery Yoga Workout

recovery

YOGA WORKOUT by DAREBEE © darebee.com

Hold each pose for 30 seconds then move on to the next one.
Repeat the sequence again on the other side.

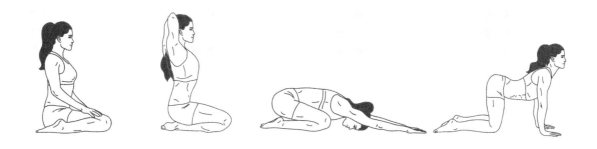

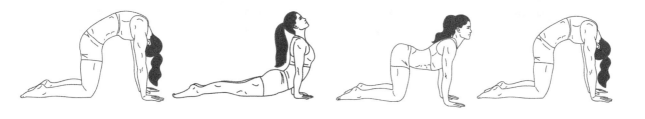

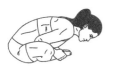 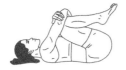 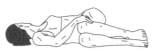 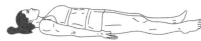

#136

Serenity Workout

SERENITY

DAREBEE WORKOUT © **darebee.com**

Hold each pose for 30 seconds then move on to the next one.
Repeat the sequence again on the other side.

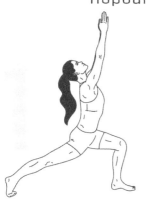 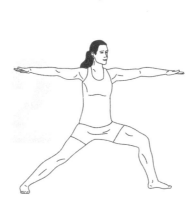 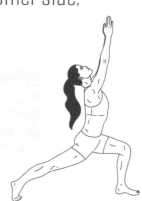

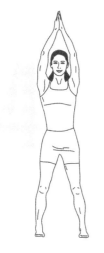 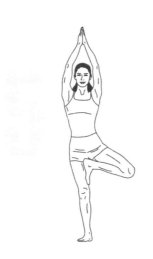 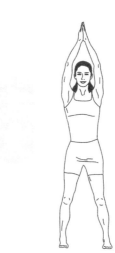

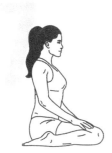 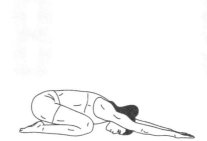 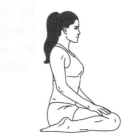

#137

Stability Workout

Stability

DAREBEE WORKOUT © darebee.com

Hold each pose for 60 seconds then move on to the next one.
30 seconds per side.

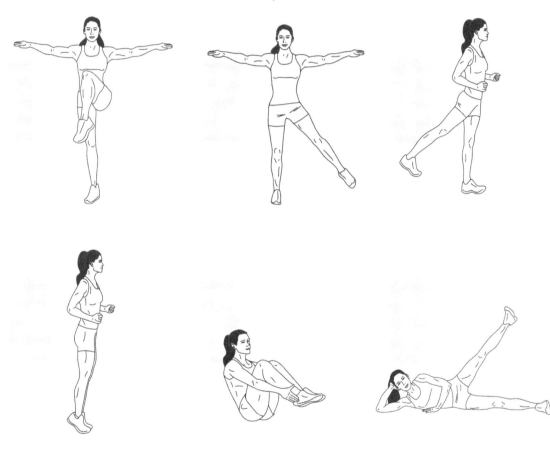

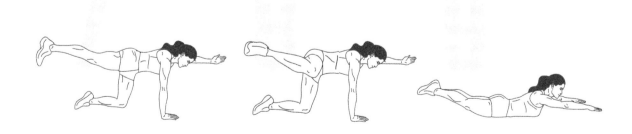

#138

Unwind Workout

UNWIND

DAREBEE WORKOUT © darebee.com

#1 Slowly shift from *Cat Pose to Cow Pose* continuously for 30 seconds.
#2 Breathe out quickly 5 times then hold the pose.
Hold each pose after #2 for 30 seconds.

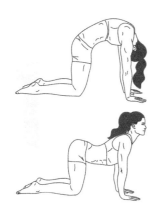
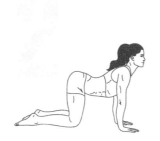
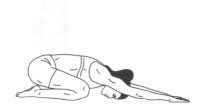

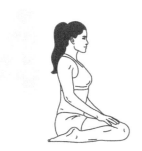
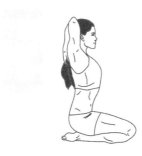
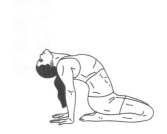

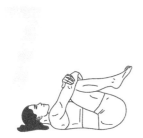
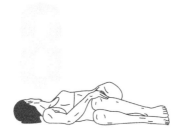
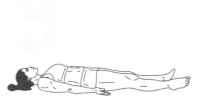

#139

Wakeup & Connect Workout

wake up
& connect

DAREBEE WORKOUT © darebee.com

Hold each pose for 20 seconds then move on to the next one.
Repeat the sequence again   on the other side.

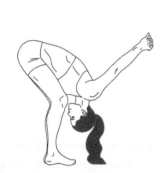
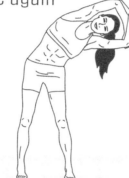
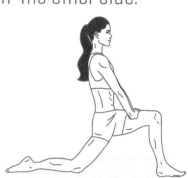

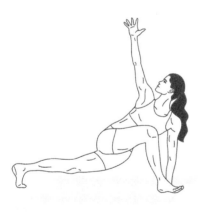
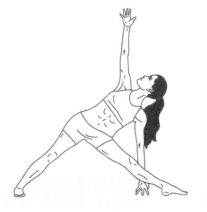
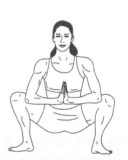

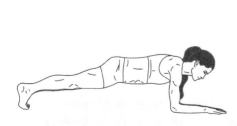
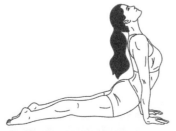
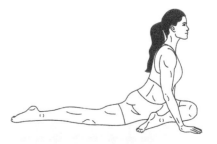

#140

Zen Workout

ZEN

DAREBEE WORKOUT © darebee.com
Hold each pose for 30 seconds then move on to the next one.

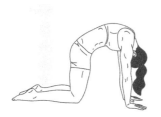 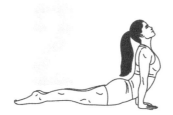 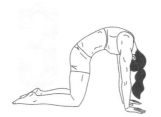

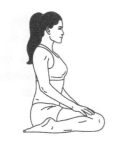 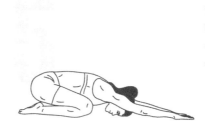 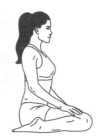

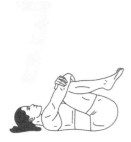 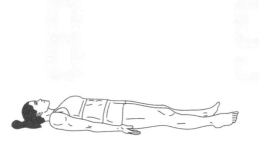 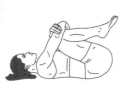

#141

2-Minute Abs Workout

2-minute abs

DAREBEE WORKOUT © darebee.com

20 seconds each exercise | no rest between exercises

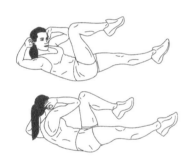

1. knee-to-elbow crunches

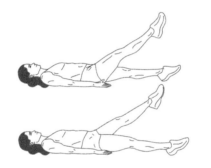

2. flutter kicks

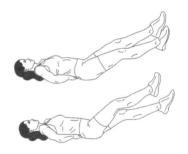

3. scissors

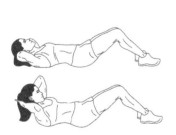

4. crunches

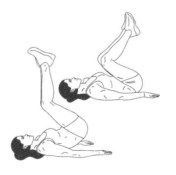

5. reverse crunches

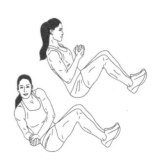

6. sitting twists

#142

Abs Defined Workout

abs defined

DAREBEE WORKOUT © darebee.com

LEVEL I 3 sets **LEVEL II** 4 sets **LEVEL III** 5 sets **REST** up to 2 minutes

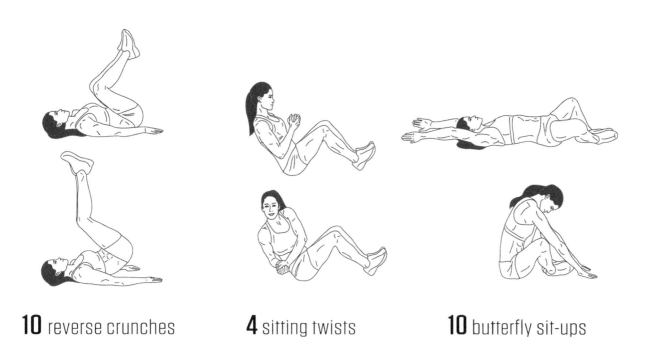

10 reverse crunches   **4** sitting twists   **10** butterfly sit-ups

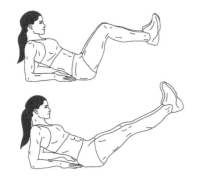   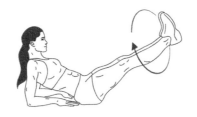   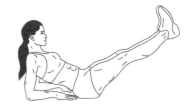

10 crunch kicks   **4** raised leg circles   **10-count** raised leg hold

#143

Anywhere Abs Workout

anywhere
abs

DAREBEE WORKOUT © darebee.com

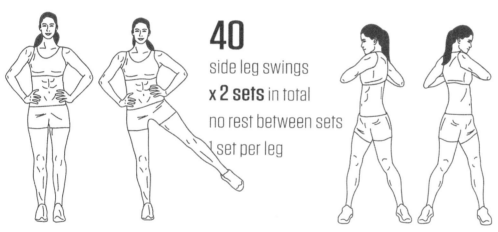

40
side leg swings
x 2 sets in total
no rest between sets
1 set per leg

10
twists
x 4 sets in total
20 seconds rest
in between sets

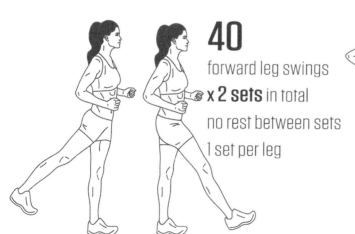

40
forward leg swings
x 2 sets in total
no rest between sets
1 set per leg

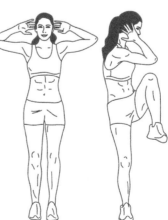

10
knee-to-elbows
x 4 sets in total
20 seconds rest
in between sets

#144

At-Home Abs Workout

at-home abs

DAREBEE WORKOUT © darebee.com

LEVEL I 3 sets **LEVEL II** 4 sets **LEVEL III** 5 sets

REST up to 2 minutes

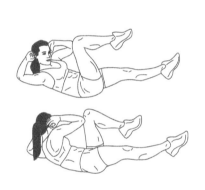

10 knee-to-elbow crunches

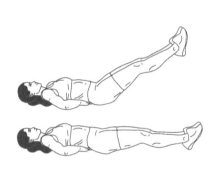

8 leg raises

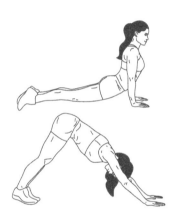

8 upward downward dog

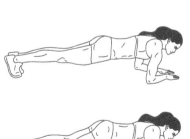
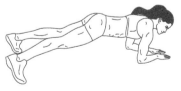

10 elbow plank step-outs

8 side plank rotations

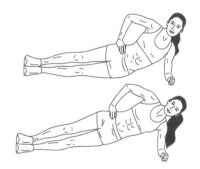

8 side bridges

#145

Chair Abs Workout

chair abs

DAREBEE WORKOUT © darebee.com

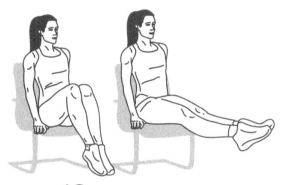

10 crunch kicks

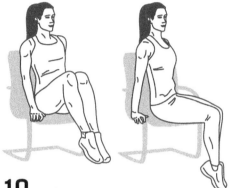

10 side-to-side knee sweeps

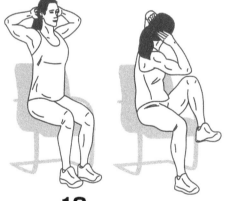

10 knee-to-elbows

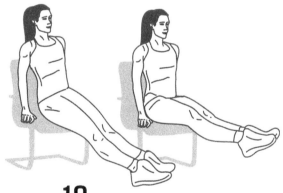

10 leg raises

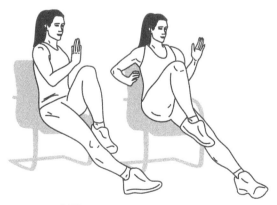

10 cycling crunches

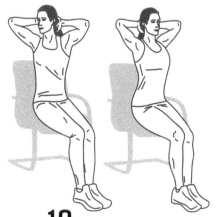

10 sitting twists

#146

Daily Abs Workout

daily abs

DAREBEE WORKOUT © darebee.com

2 minutes rest between exercises

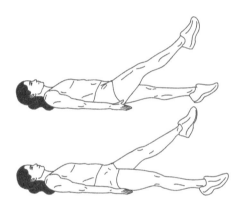

20 flutter kicks
x 3 sets in total
20 seconds rest between sets

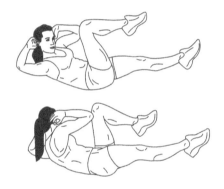

20 knee-to-elbow crunches
x 3 sets in total
20 seconds rest between sets

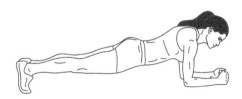

1 minutes elbow plank

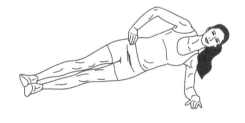

1 minutes side elbow plank
30 seconds per side

#147

Extra Crunch Workout

EXTRA CRUNCH

DAREBEE WORKOUT © darebee.com

Repeat 3 times in total

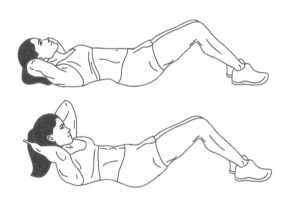

30sec crunches

30sec rest

30sec crunches

30sec rest

30sec crunches

30sec rest

30sec crunches

60sec rest

#148

Superplank Workout

super plank

DAREBEE WORKOUT © darebee.com

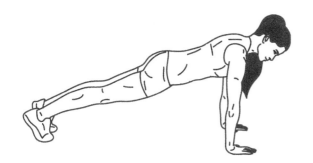

30sec plank

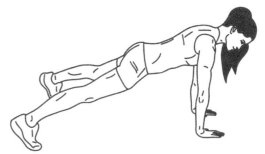

30sec wide leg plank

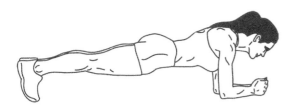

30sec elbow plank

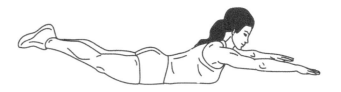

30sec superman plank

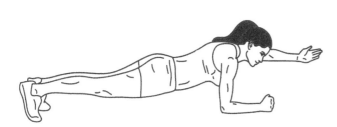

60sec raised arm elbow plank
30 seconds - each arm

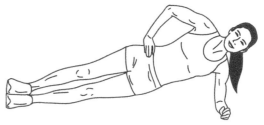

60sec side plank
30 seconds - each side

#149

Tough Cookie Workout

TOUGH COOKIE

DAREBEE WORKOUT © darebee.com

LEVEL I 3 sets **LEVEL II** 4 sets **LEVEL III** 5 sets **REST** up to 2 minutes

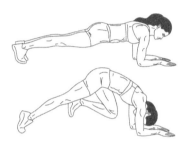

12 plank knee-ins

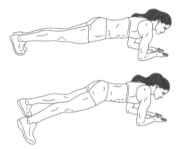

12 plank step-outs

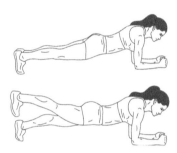

12 plank leg raises

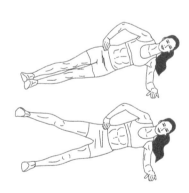

12 side plank leg raises

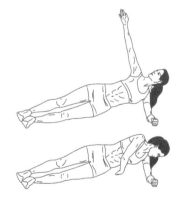

12 side plank rotations

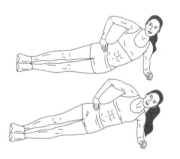

12 side bridges

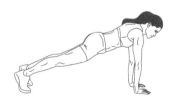
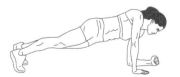
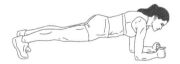

6 up and down planks

#150

Verity Workout

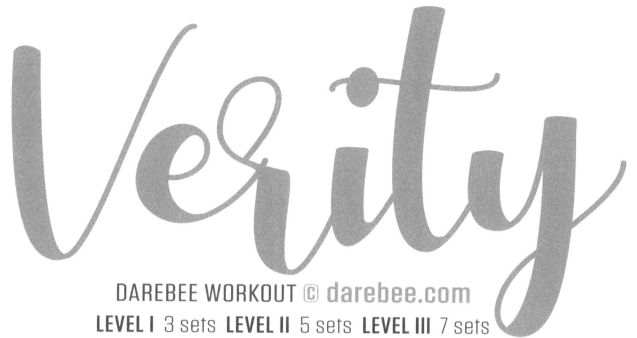

Verity

DAREBEE WORKOUT © darebee.com

LEVEL I 3 sets **LEVEL II** 5 sets **LEVEL III** 7 sets

up to 2 minutes rest between sets

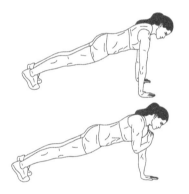

10 shoulder taps

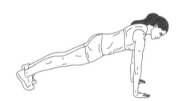

10-count plank hold

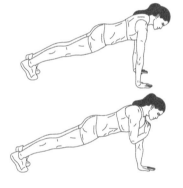

10 shoulder taps

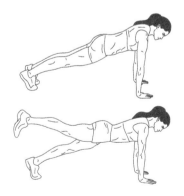

10 plank leg raises

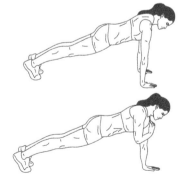

10 shoulder taps

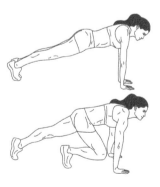

10 slow climbers

Page left blank by design

Page left blank by design.

Lightning Source UK Ltd.
Milton Keynes UK
UKHW050626240322
400554UK00007B/463